MISSION
NUTRITION

CALORIES MATTER
BUT THEY DON'T COUNT...
AT LEAST NOT THE WAY YOU THINK THEY DO

SUSAN E. SPEAR, B.S. FOOD SCIENCE, M.S. NUTRITION

nutritious

Mission Nutrition

For information about this title or to order other books and/or electronic media, contact the publisher:
Nutritious Insight, LLC
2473 S Higley Rd, Ste 104-408
Gilbert, AZ 85295
www.nutritiousinsight.com

ISBN: 978-0-9993715-1-0 (hardcover)
        978-0-9993715-2-7 (softcover)
        978-0-9993715-3-4 (ebook)

Printed in the United States of America
Cover and Interior design: 1106 Design

To my husband, Chris, for encouraging me and supporting me through Life's journey, and my mother, who continually believes in what I do. Her gentle reminder that I "needed" to write a book has echoed in my mind for many years, and I am grateful to have finally honored her request.

CONTENTS

FOREWORD   vii

INTRODUCTION: Why the Food We Eat Does More
    than Just Fill Our Stomachs   1

SECTION 1: Why Take the Journey to Making
Calories Matter?   **5**

    CHAPTER 1: Nobody Doesn't Eat   7

    CHAPTER 2: My Health Journey and
        Transformation   11

SECTION 2: The "Rules of the Road" for Making
Calories Matter   **19**

    CHAPTER 3: Stop Counting Calories—
        Learn the Truth!   21

    CHAPTER 4: Why Does Food Feel So
        Complicated?   29

    CHAPTER 5: How is My Body the Ultimate Food
        Processor?   39

SECTION 3: Taking the Journey to Transform Your
Health—Where Am I, and How Can I Get There?   **53**

CHAPTER 6: Unlocking the Secrets to Health
Transformation: Using Food to Your Advantage   55

CHAPTER 7: Commit! to Feeding Yourself with
Purpose   75

SECTION 4: Tools for the Journey to Make
Calories Matter   **91**

CHAPTER 8: What Provides the Calories in
Our Diet?   93

CHAPTER 9: Fat is Your Friend   97

CHAPTER 10: Carbohydrates Count in
Different Ways!   111

CHAPTER 11: Protein Provides   119

CHAPTER 12: What Doesn't Provide Calories in
Our Diet?   125

CHAPTER 13: Feeding Your Health
Transformation   131

CHAPTER 14: Conclusion   135

CHAPTER 15: Recipes for Success   137

ENDNOTES   141

ADDITIONAL RESOURCES   147

SUPPLEMENTAL MATERIAL   153

FOREWORD

I HAVE KNOWN SUSAN for some time now and have truly grown to appreciate her passion and dedication to discovering and sharing true principles. When something in my life isn't going well (whether in a relationship, finances, or health), I've learned that a return to true principles always has the power to lead me to significant, life-changing improvements.

For example, years ago my husband and I faced some difficult financial challenges. We worked multiple jobs, and I was thrilled to find discarded food at offices we cleaned each night. Eventually, we discovered some previously unknown-to-us principles that govern prosperity. Once we understood the principles and began to consciously live by them, we tripled our income in three months, and I became an award-winning, best-selling author, helping tens of thousands of other people experience the same kind of shift.

Just as it was with our finances, significant life-changing improvements with one's *health* also begin with a paradigm shift. When your perspective changes and you *understand the problem differently,* you feel empowered, motivated, and inspired to take the steps that lead to success. That is what this book will do for you: it will give you a new paradigm that will empower, motivate, and inspire.

I originally devoured the message in these pages because I was looking for answers to help my daughter with a newly diagnosed autoimmune disorder. I'm always amazed but never surprised when the people and resources I need show up in my life just when I need them, and the knowledge Susan has given me through this book is no exception.

As you'll soon discover, what has perhaps seemed difficult can become simple. What once seemed scary can become enjoyable. What seemed impossible can become *probable.* A slimmer waistline and better health may be closer than you think.

So, if you're like the millions of Americans who struggle with their weight or constantly battle aches, pains, and illness, *there is hope.*

And the author says it best, "In an unprecedented way, we are never without food. And yet we are malnourished and sick… When we understand the food environment, how our bodies use food, and how to eat both emotionally and physically to maximize our body's biochemistry, we have the power to reverse this trend and reclaim our future."

Let the journey begin!

— Leslie Householder
Award-winning, best-selling author of
The Jackrabbit Factor, Hidden Treasures: Heaven's Astonishing Help with Your Money Matters, and *Portal to Genius*

WHY THE FOOD WE EAT DOES MORE THAN JUST FILL OUR STOMACHS

THE STEAM RISES AS THE batter dribbles onto the pan. Cinnamon sweetness, unencumbered by kitchen walls, quickly travels through the air, inviting and enticing the sleepy-eyed dreamers away from their beds. It's Saturday morning, and the pancakes are cooking. Warm syrup simmers on the stove. Berries and bananas await. It is a ritual we never tire of. It is what we do every week. It is nourishment, it is delicious, it is love.

Go back to a time when you were with your family, eating. Was it a holiday, a dinner, a birthday celebration, a special occasion? Did you have a favorite meal or food tradition? Did you serve a food that celebrated your family's heritage? Was there a communal meal, or was it a microwave dinner of your choice, eaten "on the go"?

What are you feeling right now? Is there happy nostalgia, connection to family, a pleasant desire to have a particular food now? Or is there a feeling of anxiety, loneliness, craving, and disconnection?

Food does more than fill our stomach. It generates deep emotion. It tells our story. It creates traditions, comforts, and celebrates. It is the stuff of love, desire, connection, and nourishment to body and soul. Your food story feeds your soul.

Food also has the power to fundamentally alter how we experience health and disease, express our genes, and engage in the world around us. When we understand just how powerful food is, we can utilize it to generate meaningful transformation in our health, such as creating sustainable weight loss, helping reverse chronic health conditions, and enjoying optimal health. Transforming health begins with freeing yourself from false beliefs about willpower and counting calories. It's about busting the myth that "eating less and exercising more" is the key to losing weight and achieving health. Transforming health is achieved by knowing the "rules of the road" for eating well and making calories matter.

And that is what this book will address. This book is divided into four sections. In Section 1, I'll describe the problem with eating today and why we need to take the journey to eating well and making calories matter. I also describe my own Health Journey and Transformation. In Section 2, I'll discuss the "rules of the road" for understanding food in the grocery store and food in our bodies, and how to make sense of scientific studies. In Section 3, the journey to health transformation begins by locating where you are in the journey and helping you identify your health destination. Section 4 will provide the tools for the journey to make your calories matter by providing reliable information about food so you can make reliable decisions about what you eat. I've also included three easy recipes to help you kick-start your journey. It's time to make calories matter and learn the truth about food and how it works in your body. It's time to claim your optimal health.

SECTION 1

WHY TAKE THE JOURNEY TO MAKING CALORIES MATTER?

CHAPTER 1
NOBODY DOESN'T EAT

FOOD IS A RELATIONSHIP

OUR RELATIONSHIP WITH FOOD will be the longest relationship we'll ever have. From the day we're born until the day we die, food helps us grow, connect, and survive. Nobody doesn't eat. It is the universal experience that reminds us we are all human. It will certainly save us from death at its most basic function. Yet food is so much more than survival. It can provide powerful emotional experiences that can bring comfort, security, and well-being. But food can also become a vehicle of sadness, isolation, and illness. And food can kill us. It all depends on how we understand and manage this relationship.

EATING

Eating is simply the act of consuming food. It is influenced by geography, financial status, emotional status, the status of world peace or conflict, health status, personal preferences, and peer pressure. But physically speaking, eating is THE way we gain access to the stuff that our body needs to live. Eating is the mechanism which provides energy and essential nutrients that help us grow and thrive. The common wisdom seems to be that eating enough and eating regularly will allow survival and reproduction. Based on the world's population, we've done a pretty good job of it. It seems simple enough: If you have daily access to clean food and water—and eat it—you will live.

But something strange is happening with the health and survival of populations around the world. The good news is that infectious disease is no longer the #1 concern of the World Health Organization in developing countries.[1] The bad news is that "affluent" chronic diseases like heart disease and diabetes, usually associated with First World nations, are quickly claiming the health and economic well-being of developing nations. And it's happened in one generation. For the first time in recorded history, the upcoming generation is not expected to live as long as their parents.[2] Not only is life expectancy decreasing, but quality-of-life issues are a major economic concern since these chronic diseases severely compromise health and function and are expensive to treat long before causing death.

Chronic lifestyle-driven illnesses that used to be seen in the elderly are now occurring in younger and younger populations. What used to be called adult onset diabetes—because it mostly affected middle-aged and older adults—is now called type 2 diabetes and is regularly being diagnosed in young adults and even in the pediatric population. According to the Centers for Disease Control, type 2 diabetes has increased fourfold since 1980 from 5 million to more than 22 million Americans in 2014. Heart disease and cancer are on the rise as well. We are overweight yet undernourished. We are not starving in the traditional sense, but we are malnourished in a way never before encountered in world history.

So what is happening? Why are so many of us overweight and undernourished? Look no further for answers than the food label on that attractively packaged snack item you just purchased. The types of food we consume today are different than in the past, often containing an abundance of calories, especially from refined carbohydrates. Much of the food is highly processed, meaning it is significantly changed from its original form and nutritional content. These processed foods lack the fiber and nutrients of the original food, despite being enriched with vitamins or minerals after processing. They can also be filled with preservatives and sweeteners as well, both natural and artificial, and lots of ingredients meant to improve texture, increase flavor, and make colors more enticing. In a word, processed food is "supercharged" in every sensory category for maximum pleasure. In the food industry, these types of food are known as "highly palatable." And while these foods can feel like a "party in the mouth," they can have a serious impact on our nutrition.

We also have more access to food everywhere we go—even at gas stations. And this food is cheap. Oversized portions are an even better bargain. The average American consumer today spends less than 10% of income to obtain food, when, a generation ago, it took more than 17% of the average family's income.[3] With access to a 24/7 food environment that is cheap, abundant, and convenient, nobody can't afford to eat—generally speaking. And many can't seem to stop eating in an environment of instant access with messages about how food can make you "happy." In an unprecedented way, we are never without food. And yet we are malnourished and sick. This rapid shift in health status, occurring in one generation, needs to be clearly understood for what it is—a crisis of consumption. This is not a genetic shift but a cultural one.

The good news? When we understand the food environment, how our bodies use food, and how to eat both emotionally and physically to maximize our body's biochemistry, we have the power to reverse this trend and reclaim our future.

CHAPTER 2

MY HEALTH JOURNEY
AND TRANSFORMATION

I AM NO STRANGER TO THE chemistry and the interaction of the human body with food. My professional training includes both a bachelor's degree in food science and a master's degree in nutrition, as well as teaching both biology and nutrition at the collegiate level. As an experienced nutrition professor, I continually study the latest information in my field and actively seek to apply it to improve my own nutrition. With this background, it might seem like my health has always been on track—nutritionally speaking—but life is always more complicated, and so was my health. And I would like to share my story.

My early twenties were full of the business of being a young college graduate, working, and being a newlywed. Applying my professional understanding of food science and nutrition to my personal life over the years seemed natural. We faithfully followed the basic food groups and then the new food pyramid to guide our carbohydrate, fat, and protein intake. I paid close attention to the government Recommended Daily Allowance (now known as the Daily Reference Intake) to ensure adequate vitamin and mineral intake, and I exercised, but my health was declining, even in my twenties.

In my mid-twenties, my first child was born without complication, but I had suffered with extreme morning sickness during the entire pregnancy, and it felt like it took a long time to feel well again. A couple of years later, I had a miscarriage and serious blood loss, resulting in bone resorption and spontaneous stress fractures in my feet. Then diagnoses of endometriosis and recurring ovarian cysts were revealed, followed by two more miscarriages and surgeries. Finally, after a complicated pregnancy, in which an infection had induced pre-term labor and placed me on bed rest, my second child was born. Within six weeks of giving birth, my foot stress-fractured again. Two months later, I began experiencing debilitating abdominal pain that was diagnosed as a stomach ulcer. I was given prescription antacids and told to reduce my stress, but the pain continued, and the attacks increased in frequency. It took three months before I ended up in the emergency room, where an ultrasound finally revealed the real issue—gallstones. My gallbladder was promptly removed, and the pain finally stopped. Although "recovered," I didn't feel well much of the time despite my efforts to "eat well" and exercise.

By my mid-thirties, I was suffering from various conditions, including chronic sinus infections, sinus headaches, urinary tract infections, vertigo, unexplained skin rashes, brain fog, and excessive fatigue. This was in addition to the usual colds and flus, which constantly plagued me. I had always been tall and slender but was gaining weight and felt inflammation throughout my body. After visiting specialists, who found nothing definitive, receiving sinus surgery that did not resolve my sinus issues, and taking various medications, including a daily antibiotic for the urinary tract infections, it was clear that my health was a total disaster. I was sick. This was NOT working.

One day, after yet another sick visit to my family doctor, a "new" diagnosis was offered that would change my understanding of the power of nutrition and eventually my professional direction. My doctor explained that I probably had a systemic yeast overgrowth of the organism *Candida albicans*. Other than its relationship to antibiotic use, I was unfamiliar with the other ways this can happen in the general population and was surprised at the possibility of an overgrowth in my body. At the time, this condition was understood to affect mostly cancer patients and immunocompromised individuals and was a controversial diagnosis for anyone else, but my symptoms supported a general overgrowth throughout the body. My doctor explained that, despite using fungicides for treatment, many patients struggled to truly resolve this condition. She counseled me to use my knowledge of nutrition, as she felt this would be my best hope to reclaim my well-being. This health disaster became my "wake-up call." This was the moment when my health education really began and my scientific training and nutritional background became an indispensable tool set. I had professional training, and it was time to dig deep.

I began to re-examine the basics of how the body utilizes different foods. I discovered new information about how the gut is impacted by the type of food we eat and the medications we ingest (especially antibiotics). I also came to realize that many nutritional recommendations around vitamins and minerals had less scientific basis than previously assumed, even by professionals. Yes, there is plenty of evidence about how to avoid malnutrition, but that is not the same as studying optimal nutrition. My focus shifted to understanding optimal nutrient levels and reading studies that looked at nutrition as a therapeutic tool. I began to appreciate the optimal ranges of vitamins and minerals, as well as the role of probiotics and prebiotics, as part of a healthy diet. It also became clear that probiotics and prebiotics have an essential role in recovering health after exposure to certain medications or illnesses. Although this information may seem more mainstream today, it was radical nutrition in the very recent past.

After much trial and error, I began to understand how to more fully utilize nutrition in overcoming poor health. Using powerful probiotics and dietary adjustments not only helped to combat *Candida* overgrowth but also helped rebuild my gut flora. My gut was better able to absorb nutrients and protect my body against food sensitivities often experienced when the gut is damaged. This also positively impacted my immune system. Additionally, as my understanding about the intake of carbohydrates, fats, and proteins shifted to understanding the impact of the various TYPES of carbohydrates, fats, and protein, I began to experience a shift in my health.

In the beginning, I had to eliminate certain foods, like dairy and citrus, for a period of time, but that is not uncommon with a damaged gut. Over time, my gut became more resilient, and foods that had previously caused sensitivity were reintroduced. I can once again consume dairy but only do so occasionally, as I have discovered other delicious options. I enjoy eating whole fresh citrus from our citrus trees, especially grapefruit. The most important information I encountered was the power of a diet low in sugar, especially added sugar. Understanding how the consumption of sugar can dramatically impact gut health, increase inflammation, increase metabolic dysfunction in organs, increase heart disease risk, and promote *Candida* overgrowth and cancer was more life changing for me than almost all the other information gathered.

Today, I no longer suffer with excessive and chronic fatigue, *Candida* overgrowth, sinus problems, vertigo, chronic urinary tract infections, rashes, and endometriosis, and have only the occasional headache. My feet no longer spontaneously stress-fracture, and my inflammation is subdued. My blood work is healthier than ever before. I no longer follow a food pyramid but use reliable nutrition resources and keep up with respected researchers to inform my dietary intake. I now eat in a way that supports my needs and includes a focus on low-glycemic carbohydrates, inclusion of healthy fats, and adequate protein. I have also learned the value of incorporating additional healing modalities such as acupuncture and became a master herbalist, knowledgeably utilizing herbal supplements and essential oils. Getting outside and enjoying walks and hikes with friends and family is my exercise. Most importantly, I protect myself from the avalanche of added sugar, chemical additives, and simple starches so abundant in our culture.

My health struggle has made me much more aware of what nutrition can really do, what sugar really is, and the necessity of taking responsibility for protecting my health. I no longer "outsource" my nutrition to convenience foods that appear "healthy" based on calorie count and other health claims and carefully prepare more nutritious options at home. It's not about always skipping dessert but about being aware of my sugar consumption and knowing how to celebrate without causing metabolic chaos in my body's digestion process.

Eating, in general, moves us either toward a state of health or toward a state of disease. Do our choices really have such consequences? Yes—sometimes immediately, but over time ALWAYS. We can choose to eat in opposition to our health or in support of it. It is that simple.

Is there one "perfect" diet for "perfect" health? No! But there are important basic principles for eating that make a difference in your health. What follows is a proven pathway to health transformation.

First, we need to understand what a calorie really is and what eating a calorie really does.

The next step may seem obvious, but it's often ignored. In order to begin the journey to better health and nutrition, we need to know where we presently stand nutritionally.

Is our diet adequate? Is it lacking in a particular vitamin or mineral? How much fat, carbohydrate, and protein are regularly consumed? We benefit from obtaining relevant blood tests (beyond the cholesterol panel) and should consider a genetic evaluation in order to gain more information about how we might optimally support our wellness.

Finally, we need to gain a basic understanding of what food is and how to utilize it to our advantage. We need to become aware of physical, emotional, and psychological cues to our eating patterns and honor our food relationship. By working with our food, our emotions, and our environment, we can work with our bodies. Life can be lived deliciously with a body prepared to function optimally over a lifetime.

SECTION 2

THE "RULES OF THE ROAD" FOR MAKING CALORIES MATTER

CHAPTER 3

STOP COUNTING CALORIES— LEARN THE TRUTH!

HOW DOES A CALORIE ACTUALLY COUNT?

CALORIES REPRESENT ENERGY from food. We need calories from food to supply our body with energy to function. Our brain, breathing, digestion, circulation, and cell repair all require a basic number of calories. This survival level of energy is known as the basal metabolic rate (BMR). Any extra energy required for activity and self-care such as eating, walking, showering, and exercising requires additional calories. If someone consumes an excess number of calories, they will potentially store them as fat. If fewer calories are consumed, stored energy can be used, and weight loss may occur.

How many calories do we need? Well, it is not a "static" number and changes daily. So here are some basics about calorie requirements: Gender affects caloric need. Age affects caloric need. Size (height and bone mass) affects caloric need.

If you have more lean body mass (muscle), you will have a higher basal metabolic rate and burn more calories. Illness and physical stress can increase caloric need. Men generally require more calories than women. Elite athletes need to consume a lot more calories than a non-athlete would consume. No two people will have exactly the same caloric needs. A person's caloric needs will also vary each day due to different activities and stress. Are you beginning to see that daily calorie needs can vary in many ways? There's no question that we need a significant number of calories, generally no less than 1,500 and upwards of 2,500 per day, to maintain health, but we won't "need" exactly the same number of calories each day. Fortunately, our bodies can successfully navigate this variation and maintain a healthy weight range if we understand how calories work.

Calorie counting to achieve an "ideal" weight has been the focus of what we culturally understand about calories in the last thirty years. We assume that a "thin" individual is a healthy individual. We also assume that weight is an accurate indicator of our state of health. So it's easy to adopt the "logic" that simply accounting for the number of calories that corresponds to height and activity level will inevitably produce a desirable weight and state of health in anyone who is motivated and willing to do the work. This is reinforced by recent advice given to consumers from a national beverage association that says that all calories count, regardless of where they come from. This is correct: Calories count. But this is also incomplete. It's time to understand the whole story.

It's true that fat, carbohydrates, and protein have different calorie counts to be accounted for, and this fact may cause you to assume that eating fat versus a carbohydrate will cause more weight gain because fat has more calories. Or you may have heard that eating high protein, low fat, and low carb is the way to go. But this is only one part of the story. Acknowledging the significant increase in obesity and chronic disease just in the United States in the last generation despite using the "logic" of calorie counting clearly indicates a problem with just counting calories. Simply adding up calories from each of the fat, carbohydrate and protein groups to arrive at the "right" number of calories to match energy expenditure for the day and maintain an "ideal weight" and potentially improve health isn't working. It isn't just calories in, calories out. It isn't always about eating less if you want to lose weight and "be healthy." It isn't about exercising more to compensate for "extra" calories if you want dessert. The story of calorie inequality goes much deeper.

The type of calorie, or where it comes from, is more important than the number of calories. Not all calories are equal when it comes to how your body processes them. It is about understanding HOW our bodies process calories once they are consumed. This is POWERFUL information that will allow you to maximize your nutritional efforts.

Take carbohydrates, for example. What a carbohydrate calorie does in the body can vary tremendously. It isn't just about carbs, fats, and proteins. It's about the TYPE of carb, fat, and protein. The real answer lies within the biochemical processes in your body. For example, carbohydrates can either promote abdominal fat or encourage a leaner body—even when the SAME number of calories is eaten. Consuming 200 calories from a fruit juice is not the same as consuming 200 calories from raw fruits or vegetables. Even though all of these 200 calorie items are carbohydrates, they will process very differently in the body and produce different fat storage and nutritional signals.

HOW OATMEAL HELPED A HARVARD PROFESSOR

I like to refer to the story of oatmeal and a frustrated Harvard professor from the book *Always Hungry*, by Dr. David Ludwig, when discussing the idea of calorie inequality and why simple calorie counting doesn't work for weight management. Back in the mid 1990s, Dr. David Ludwig, today a noted Harvard professor and pediatric endocrinologist, was frustrated by the failure of his obese pediatric patients to manage their weight and health risks despite carefully counting calories and balancing fat, protein, and carbohydrate intake. Dr. Ludwig was using low-fat diets and carefully limiting calories with no success. His patients were following the "approved" diet for weight loss in the medical community, and yet it was not working. Were his patients lazy and non-compliant, or was there another reason that had nothing to do with his patients' willpower and activity level?

Nutritional dogma had taught that, as long as you accounted for a calorie as a fat, protein, or carbohydrate, no further distinction was necessary. A carb is a carb, a fat is a fat, and a protein is a protein. But this idea was failing miserably in clinical practice. Meanwhile Dr. Ludwig began to search the medical literature and found that a failure of the calorie model was not new. He came across a 1959 systemic review of thirty years of medical weight-loss programs. This exhaustive review was conducted by researchers in Philadelphia and New York, and it concluded that medical weight-loss programs did not work. Thirty years of studies showed that counting calories did not work for sustained weight loss or weight control! Additional review of the literature from the 1980s continued to show that counting calories was ineffective for long-term weight management. Strangely, this data was generally disregarded in clinical recommendations, and the calories in = calories out model continued to be foundational in nutrition and weight-management recommendations. Patients were told to eat less and exercise more to satisfy this type of weight-loss model, yet the literature clearly demonstrated that this idea was flawed.

Curious to test a different approach to how we think about calories, Dr. Ludwig conducted a groundbreaking study in the mid 1990s. Yes, it is a small study from the '90s, but it was one of the earliest formal attempts at challenging the idea that all calories are equal and that eating a processed cereal from a whole grain is no different metabolically than eating that same number of calories from an unprocessed whole grain or animal protein. Dr. Ludwig's study, published in the journal *Pediatrics*,[4] gave twelve adolescent boys three different breakfasts following an overnight stay in a metabolic ward at the hospital. All three breakfasts had the SAME number of calories, but the amount and type of carbohydrate varied among them. One breakfast was "instant" oatmeal, a highly processed carbohydrate. Although a whole grain by definition, instant oatmeal has been pulverized into small pieces and cooked at a high temperature prior to packaging. This type of carbohydrate will pass quickly into the bloodstream and produce a rapid and significant rise in blood sugar and insulin (a high glycemic index and load). The second breakfast was steel-cut oats, considered a minimally processed carbohydrate. This time, the whole-grain label is more obvious since the kernel is left mostly intact. This larger, more-intact kernel takes longer to cook, but it also takes longer to digest than the instant oats and produces a smaller rise in glucose and insulin. Both oat "meals" had the same nutrients of about 65% carbohydrate, 20% fat. The third breakfast was a vegetable omelet with fruit. This had more protein and fat, less carbohydrate, and no grains, but it still had the same number of calories as the other two breakfasts.

The initial blood glucose and insulin results were not a total surprise. Blood sugar and insulin levels initially went up to high, intermediate, and low levels based on the first, second, and third type of breakfast. But what happened next was more interesting. One hour after the instant oatmeal, blood sugar fell rapidly. After four hours, it was lower than when compared to the other two meals and even lower than after the overnight fast. This drop in blood sugar was so large that the body was provoked to hunger. Unlike the other two meals, the instant oatmeal also caused free fatty acids in the blood to drop in a negative fashion, which further aggravated blood-sugar levels. Emergency stress hormones were triggered, and adrenaline surged four hours after the instant oatmeal. The body perceived this as a metabolic crisis, with participants showing signs of hypoglycemia (shaking and sweating).

These teens were then served the same meals again at lunch and then allowed to eat as much or as little as they wanted from large platters of bread, bagels, cold cuts, cream cheese, regular cheese, spreads, cookies, and fruits throughout the afternoon. The instant-oatmeal group ate substantially more calories (1,400 calories) compared to the steel-cut oats group (900 calories) and omelet-with-fruit group (750 calories). The instant-oatmeal group consumed 650 calories more during the afternoon than the omelet-and-fruit group, even though both of those meals contained the same number of calories.

What can a difference of 650 calories add up to over time? If this difference occurred day after day, it could explain much of the increase in body weight since the 1970s, as consumption of highly processed carbohydrates has skyrocketed. Meals with the same calories can produce dramatically different metabolic outcomes a few hours later. A carb isn't just a carb! The kind of oatmeal you eat matters! And managing hunger signals and weight isn't just about willpower!

There are now numerous studies demonstrating that not all types of carbohydrate calories are processed equally in the body. Prominent research has focused on sugar consumption and fructose in particular, demonstrating the profound differences in carbohydrate metabolism. Many researchers are continuing to produce high-quality, peer-reviewed, impactful studies about the significant differences among carbohydrates. I have chosen to tell the story of Dr. Ludwig, as he remains one of the premier early researchers on this topic, authoring more than one hundred peer-reviewed scientific articles.

CHAPTER 4
WHY DOES FOOD FEEL SO COMPLICATED?

PART I:
FOOD "RULES" AND FOOD SCIENCE

THIS SECTION IS ABOUT understanding a few basic American "food rules" and quirks around how we label and evaluate the food we eat. It's just an explanation of what Americans, by law, have immediate access to when they purchase a food product. It is ONE way to understand our diet. It is also helpful to have just a little bit of background in the science of food so you can gain more confidence in understanding your diet.

FOOD LABELS IN AMERICA
The food label, or Nutrition Facts Label, gives us information about fat, protein, and carbohydrates and a few vitamins

and minerals, so we can understand the source of our calories. For example, a label might state that one serving has 4.5 grams of fat and that this is 7% of your daily value for fat calories based on a 2,000-calorie-per-day diet. If enough of this information is recorded during the day, it is possible to determine the overall composition of your diet. Calories eaten that day could be composed of 20% protein, 40% carbs, and 40% fat. It is also possible to determine certain micronutrient information, such as your sodium or vitamin A intake and learn what percentage of the government-recommended intake is being met by that food. But food labels are only one aspect of understanding a healthy diet. They do not contain all the information you need to build a healthy diet. And they are not always easy to understand, given that serving sizes may not match your actual intake, and the number of calories in your diet may vary from the 2,000 calories used in computing percentages of intake. It requires more than a quick glance to effectively read and use a Nutrition Facts Label.

TRICKY BUT TRUE FACT ABOUT FOOD LABELS
The 0.5 gram rule and the Nutrition Facts Label
The FDA allows food manufacturers to list an ingredient as 0 grams on the Nutrition Facts Label if the serving size contains less than 0.5 grams. If you eat multiple servings of something that lists 0 grams on the label but actually contains 0.4 grams/serving, you will be ingesting a measurable amount. This applies to sugar, fat, trans-fats, protein, and carbohydrates.

UNDERSTANDING "ORGANIC"

The term "organic" can seem like a simple, straightforward way to evaluate food—and it is, when applied correctly. Today, an "organic" label indicates that a food was produced with little or no synthetic pesticides and no antibiotics or hormones. "Organic" labeling guidelines are established by the USDA and focus on how a particular food item was farmed or raised. It is important to understand what the term "organic" does and does NOT mean in the United States. The term "organic" is NOT a reliable indicator of the vitamin and mineral content of food and does not serve as a guideline for evaluating the nutritional content, safety, or quality of a product. It also does not indicate the amount of processing the food has undergone.

The original idea behind the organic movement was that the soil should be conserved, protected, and regenerated, and this became the basis for the USDA Organic Food Production Act, passed in 1990. These guidelines established four basic standards of organic foods: (1) a national certification program for production, (2) an official USDA label for products, (3) a national list of approved and prohibited substances such as pesticides and fertilizers for organic production, and (4) an accreditation program for agents who would certify a producer's compliance with organic production standards. Animal-welfare standards were added later, along with exclusion of certain technologies, such as irradiation—a practice common in the spice industry—and genetically modified organisms (GMOs). Again, "organic" does not indicate that cattle are grass-fed or chickens are pasture-raised. It's interesting to note that highly processed foods, such as cheese curls, can be considered "organic" but are not considered a nutrient-dense, optimal snack food. Remember, "organic" does not consider the nutritional content of a food or its quality and safety.

How do you determine if a product is organic? It's easy to identify a single item of produce as 100% organic, but what happens when a product has a lot of ingredients? In order for a product to qualify for the official USDA organic seal on its label, at least 95% of the ingredients must be organic. These products may prominently display the green and white USDA "organic" seal. If the product contains at least 70% organic ingredients, the label can prominently display "Made with Organic _____," but cannot carry the USDA organic seal anywhere. If the product contains less than 70% organic ingredients, the label can use the word "organic" to identify only specific components in the ingredient list.[5]

Should you buy only products with the USDA organic seal? Is the official USDA organic "seal" the only way to identify a responsibly and sustainably farmed or raised food product? As a consumer, you do not have to rely on the USDA organic seal label as the only way to identify pesticide-free, GMO-free, antibiotic-free, and hormone-free food. A responsible farmer and food producer will clearly label their products as antibiotic free, GMO-free, or pesticide free and encourage the consumer to look into their production methods. In fact, some producers do not consider the organic label as relevant or selective enough to promote their overall mission of creating both sustainable AND nutritious, high-quality food products.

Another thing to understand about the official USDA organic seal is that obtaining this status and label is costly and time consuming for the farmer and producer. Some small food manufacturers and producers do not have the resources to seek official organic certification or may be awaiting approval; however, their production practices may already meet or even exceed the minimum practices required to be considered "organic." This creates an interesting choice for the consumer, since the product may be "organic" in every way except for the official "seal" on the label. Official labels can promote confidence and trust, but in the end, the environmentally responsible manufacturers and producers can still clearly label their products with their farming practices and organic ingredients and can provide every assurance of sustainable farming practices even without the official USDA organic seal. And if you are lucky enough to buy your products directly from the farmer or producer, you can see for yourself how they produce their products.

HOW TO BE A DATA EXPERT: UNDERSTANDING THE DATA DRAMA

Epidemiological Studies *vs.* Clinical Studies

One challenge commonly encountered in science is how to interpret and utilize data collected in a study. Interpreting data is both an art and a science and depends first and foremost on the type of study that is conducted. Understanding the basic design of a study profoundly impacts how data can be applied to a topic and, ultimately, your life.

Fundamentally, there are two types of studies: One is designed to identify associations or correlations and trends, as well as identify what does NOT cause something, while the other is designed to determine what DOES cause something. These are two very different capabilities of a study. The general terms for these two types of studies are epidemiological and clinical.

An interesting case history using the power of both epidemiological and clinical studies occurred in Philadelphia in 1976. A strange outbreak of pneumonia was observed among people attending the American Legion Convention in Philadelphia in 1976.[6] Epidemiologists were able to identify a variety of risk factors that were associated with the onset of pneumonia while eliminating those factors that were not. The associated risk factors were then tested in clinical laboratory settings to identify which might actually be a cause. Six months later, clinical studies were able to successfully identify one species of bacteria, Legionnaires' bacillus, as the cause of the outbreak, based on the risk factors identified in the epidemiological study.

An epidemiological study observes a population of humans or animals and then attempts to discover what risk factors are associated with a disease occurring within that population. It studies disease patterns and frequency without attempting an intervention. The findings are statistically analyzed and used to suggest a future trend for the incidence of a disease. Results from this type of study are qualitative in nature, meaning they are observational and subjective. They help develop theory.

There are a couple of challenges in designing an epidemiological or observational study. One of the challenges is to clearly define the disease being studied. The other challenge is the criterion used to classify someone as a "case" (someone with the disease) or a "control" (those without disease). By clearly defining a disease and a case, the collection of data can be more precise and strengthen the ability to find real trends and associations in a population. This can more accurately identify risk factors.

A competent researcher also carefully accounts for and limits the number of factors (variables) being studied but still endeavors to identify and enroll as many cases as possible. Accounting for and eliminating what are known as third, or confounding, variables when designing the study is important to protecting the accuracy and usefulness of the data. On the other hand, including large numbers of cases is more likely to identify a significant association between the disease and the risk factor, but only if a significant association actually exists.

A lack of correlation (association) is easier to find than strong correlation in an observational study, but both have value. A lack of correlation is valuable because it can prove that a factor does NOT contribute to or cause a disease. Ultimately, though, associations are sought, and well-designed repeated studies will identify common associations and add strength to the importance of a risk factor. Data can then be used to recommend specific control measures. But here is the catch with any epidemiological study: While it provides important understanding about association between a risk factor and a disease, it remains just that—an association. It is not causation. And this has limits in scientific circles.

An epidemiological study can NEVER prove causation. It can never prove that a particular risk factor is the actual cause of the disease or condition being studied; epidemiological studies look for trends in large populations. This type of study is fundamentally qualitative in nature and subjective. While correlation (association) can be unmistakable, with a high incidence occurring with exposure to the risk factor, there is still the possibility that an unknown factor which was not studied and happens to be associated with the studied risk factor (a potential confounding variable) is actually the cause.

A useful analogy can be found in the incidence of fires and the appearance of firemen at fires. An epidemiological study will find a strong correlation between the appearance of firemen and the incidence of fire at the same location. It might also find that the larger the fire, the larger the number of firemen. A strong association like this might persuade someone who learns of this association and who is otherwise unfamiliar with fires to conclude that, since firemen are always in attendance at a fire, they are actually causing the fires. They may also conclude that the more firemen who show up, the larger the fire will be. While the conclusions are obviously flawed and easily disproved, it is not so obvious in actual practice with epidemiological studies. This is where epidemiological studies and clinical studies come together.

Clinical studies are conducted in laboratories under controlled conditions and use quantifiable interventions based on suspected risk factors. These can be animal or human studies. Quantifiable (measurable) exposures to agents (factors) are administered during the clinical study to understand the onset or prevention of disease. Studies focus on producing or preventing a disease by intervening with a specific risk factor(s). Studies also demonstrate reliability of an outcome. Often the factor being studied has been determined by previous epidemiological studies to show a strong association between that risk factor and a disease. Clinical studies are capable of proving causation due to the application of specific controls and quantifiable interventions which have high reproducibility and demonstrate reliable outcomes.

In nutrition, it is important to combine epidemiological evidence with well-designed clinical studies to avoid "common sense" conclusions and generate measurable and reliable data about food intake, weight loss, and disease. We have seen the problem with dietary cholesterol and fat recommendations in particular when only epidemiological studies were employed as the basis for "causation" for heart disease. We have also tested the "calories in = calories out" model for weight loss against a clinical standard and found it to be a poor descriptor of how the body's biochemistry actually uses calories. In fact, clinical studies have shown that exercise is not a reliable mechanism for weight control, despite popular medical opinion.[7] Well-designed clinical studies are showing that dietary cholesterol is not a driver of heart disease and that saturated fat in the absence of refined carbohydrates raises HDL cholesterol, a good thing. Meta-analysis of epidemiological studies demonstrates a lack of correlation between saturated fat and cardiovascular disease, and that is useful because lack of correlation does prove lack of causation.

The important message about scientific studies is that there is power in cooperation between well-designed and well-conducted epidemiological and clinical studies along with a robust interpretation of these studies. All studies, both epidemiological and clinical, enable us to make ever-more-precise decisions about how we interact with the world. But we must still acknowledge our limitations. As much as we would like to claim a flawless method to correctly identify all risk factors and perfectly determine causation, it remains elusive. Science, itself, is a process for increasingly arriving at ever-more-defensible answers to our questions but rarely an unquestionable solution. While causation has been reliably determined in certain limited situations, one can also find credible studies with conflicting conclusions on many topics. The reality is that most studies will not provide the definitive answer but instead provide useful and defensible understanding on a subject that will continue to be revised as more studies provide more insight. Uncertainty remains a constant companion in research. Continuing to ask better questions, fearlessly pursuing answers, and revising conclusions and subsequent recommendations as the data informs us are our best use of science and give us our best opportunity to understand a topic and give context to the world around us.

CHAPTER 5

HOW IS MY BODY THE ULTIMATE FOOD PROCESSOR?

PART II:
BASIC HUMAN PHYSIOLOGY and FOOD

TRIGLYCERIDES—A FAT IN YOUR BLOOD

TRIGLYCERIDES, LIKE CHOLESTEROL, are a type of fat that can be found and measured in the blood. Triglycerides store unused calories, acting as an energy reservoir. The concentration of triglycerides in the blood (serum) can be highly predictive of the risk of stroke.

The interesting thing about triglycerides is that they don't come just from your diet. The body, specifically the liver, can make triglycerides. So what determines your serum-triglyceride levels? There are two types of serum-triglyceride levels, fasting and post-prandial (following a meal), and there are a couple of contributors to these levels. Although dietary fat initially raises serum triglycerides following a meal, this is a *short-term* result of the digestive process. Triglycerides from a meal quickly become "packaged" particles called chylomicrons in the intestines, get absorbed into the bloodstream, and raise serum-triglyceride levels, but then they are efficiently processed through the liver in a few hours. This dietary fat is a *minor* contributor to serum levels after a meal and does not contribute to *fasting* serum-triglyceride levels.

There are non-meal reactions that do significantly impact fasting and post-prandial serum-triglyceride levels in the body. For example, abdominal (visceral) fat is insulin resistant and ends up contributing this fat to the bloodstream by continually dumping fatty acids into the liver. Once in the liver, these fatty acids will be made into triglycerides and pushed into the bloodstream. This raises serum-triglyceride levels not only after a meal but beyond. In fact, this liver triglyceride factory will keep going as long as these fatty acids continue to pour in—24 hours a day. This is a major contributor to both post-meal and fasting serum-triglyceride levels.

One of the biggest sources of fasting serum-triglyceride levels is refined or simple carbohydrates. These types of carbohydrates will turn into saturated fat in your bloodstream via the liver, where they are converted to triglycerides and pushed into the bloodstream. These carbohydrate conversions are responsible for most of the fasting circulating-triglycerides levels.[8, 9] Fasting serum-triglyceride levels reflect carbohydrate consumption, not fat consumption.

Once again, fasting serum-triglyceride levels originate from carbohydrate consumption and from fatty acid dumping from insulin-resistant abdominal fat! I know, fat coming from carbohydrates…not from *dietary fat?* It is biochemistry in action. But the important physiological point is that fasting triglycerides above 150 mg/dL are able to provide unique information about heart disease risk and are much more predictive than total cholesterol alone ever was.[10] Ideally, triglycerides should be below 100 mg/dL. When it comes to heart disease risk, it's NOT the dietary fat, it's the refined carbohydrates!

HORMONES THAT MATTER: INSULIN, LEPTIN, AND CORTISOL

Insulin: What Is It?

Insulin is a hormone responsible for controlling the transport of glucose from the bloodstream into the fat, liver, and skeletal muscle cells. It also helps muscle cells uptake amino acids to build muscle. Insulin is important for the metabolism of carbohydrates, protein, and fats, but its predominant function involves glucose uptake and storage. Insulin is like a "key" that fits into a special insulin receptor on a cell, unlocking the cell for glucose and/or amino acids to enter. It is made in the pancreas by the beta cells and released in response to a rise of glucose or amino acids in the blood.

Yes, insulin can reduce blood sugar, but *insulin is first and foremost a storage hormone that happens to reduce blood sugar.* Its real function is to store energy (anabolic) in the body for times of scarcity, and it prefers to store it as fat. When glucose levels in the blood become elevated, insulin transports the glucose out of the bloodstream and into cells for storage. Glucose becomes converted to glycogen in the muscle cells or triglycerides in fat cells, or both in the liver. When there is more sugar in the bloodstream than is required for cellular needs, insulin will store that sugar in the liver, mostly as triglycerides (fat) and not glycogen, since glycogen storage is finite in the normal liver.

Protein and Insulin

While it's commonly understood that sugar (carbohydrate) or glucose raises insulin, protein can do it, too—especially whey protein. In normal individuals, the insulin response to protein occurs in order to promote uptake of amino acids to build and repair tissues. This insulin rise is specific to the amino-acid content and does not correlate with the increase in blood glucose that occurs from carbohydrate ingestion. When protein is eaten in excess of this need for muscle and tissue repair, the amino acids remain in the bloodstream and eventually convert to glucose. This eventually raises blood sugar, and insulin will no longer transport amino acids but instead transport excess blood sugar into cells for storage— mostly as fat.

In appropriate amounts, the body can fully utilize amino acids from a protein meal to build muscle, and this insulin reaction can be beneficial to build bulk. However, once the muscles have enough amino acids, they won't continue to uptake any more amino acids. These excess amino acids will become excess blood sugar and be stored as fat. This can explain why excess milk consumption can cause rapid weight gain, including in bottle-fed infants.

Milk and Insulin: A Special Case

There is also interesting interaction between protein and carbohydrates and insulin release. When protein is consumed in conjunction with carbohydrates, it will raise insulin levels even higher than if the intake were just carbohydrates (glucose) alone. Milk is a particularly powerful trigger for raising insulin in many people due to the combination of its carbohydrate and whey protein content. This is due to whey's high content of branched-chain amino acids, which absorb rapidly—NOT the lactose (sugar) content of milk. Milk can produce a three- to six-fold increase in the insulinemic response compared to the same amount of glucose.[11]

Why We Love Insulin

Without proper insulin levels, our cells are unable to absorb glucose or amino acids from the bloodstream, and this is life threatening—so insulin is vital to life. But it is important for insulin to remain within a healthy range, and cells need to remain sensitive to insulin signals; otherwise, there is metabolic chaos. Metabolic chaos commonly includes insulin resistance.

Insulin Resistance and Development of Type 2 Diabetes

Insulin resistance is a condition in which cells or organs are not responding to insulin's signals. This condition does not develop all at once in every cell or organ, but sequentially. The liver becomes resistant first, followed by muscle tissue, and then fat cells. When you wake up in the morning and blood sugar is already high, it's because the resistant liver isn't responding to insulin's signal to stop making and releasing sugar (glucose) into the bloodstream. And this extra sugar can't be properly accepted and "burned" by the resistant muscle tissue, either. So the liver is producing glucose, and the muscle can't use it; this raises blood sugar. The fat cells will continue to be insulin sensitive and continue taking in this sugar and storing it as fat, increasing body weight. Eventually weight gain plateaus as even the fat cells become insulin resistant.

When the liver, muscle, and fat cells become insulin resistant, the pancreas will try to produce even more insulin in an effort to overwhelm the cells with opportunities to take up the circulating blood sugar. Insulin is circulating all of the time. High levels of circulating insulin are a signal that metabolism is dysfunctional. Cell communication is disrupted, and, eventually, disease results, including type 2 diabetes, which includes not only insulin resistance but consistently high blood-sugar levels.

Why Insulin Resistance?

As we age, repeated cellular exposure to insulin produces resistance at some level, and this cannot be completely stopped. However, we can potentially influence the *rate* at which insulin resistance occurs in the cell by controlling the diet. Excessive intakes of sugar in the diet increase insulin levels and expose cells to increased sugar uptake. Cells are able to store only a certain amount of sugar and eventually reduce the number of insulin receptors on their membrane as a protection from too much sugar, and this is insulin resistance. A diet high in sugar and non-fibrous carbohydrates requires more insulin to metabolize the sugar, increasing the frequency that the cell gets exposed to insulin and increasing the rate at which insulin resistance develops. Lowering sugar intake and increasing dietary fiber reduces spikes in blood sugar and chronic exposure to high levels of insulin, potentially mediating development of insulin resistance.

And "sugar" does not refer only to glucose when it comes to insulin resistance. It also refers to fructose and galactose, which will also indirectly provoke insulin resistance. Fructose is particularly problematic in this regard. All simple sugars promote insulin resistance. And insulin resistance promotes more insulin production in a vicious cycle for the pancreas. High levels of insulin can overwhelm the least-resistant cells to uptake sugar at some level, but this is not sustainable for the pancreas or the cells. The pancreas will not be able to continue to increase insulin production indefinitely. Cells will not be able to take in the increasing amount of sugar from the bloodstream. Eventually, blood sugar will become chronically elevated, a sign of diabetes.

The Insulin Avalanche

What do high levels of circulating insulin do to the body? Insulin causes cellular proliferation, including a build-up of plaque by stimulating endothelial proliferation. Insulin also causes the blood to clot too readily and causes macrophages (immune cells) to accumulate as fatty deposits. This is cardiovascular disease. Cancer is also stimulated by excess insulin—cancer cells are known to have receptors for insulin and insulin-like growth factors. Excess insulin causes excretion of magnesium and calcium in the urine, leading to osteoporosis. Excess insulin can also cause the calcium, if it isn't excreted, to wander around (no longer receiving proper instruction from the anabolic hormones in your insulin-resistant tissues) and deposit in the wrong places. Instead of building bone, it will create calcifications everywhere, including the arteries and kidneys. In summary, elevated insulin is highly associated and even causative for several diseases: heart disease, peripheral vascular disease, stroke, high blood pressure, kidney stones, cancer, obesity, osteoporosis, and other metabolic disorders.

The Appetite Factor: Leptin

Leptin is a hormone secreted by adipose (fat) tissue. Leptin is the way that fat cells communicate with the brain about how much energy is on board and how that energy should be used. It sends a powerful signal to the brain that regulates appetite, fat storage, maintenance and repair of tissues, and whether you should reproduce (puberty). Overall, leptin functions to decrease appetite. When fat cells are "full," extra fat will cause a surge in leptin, signaling the brain to stop feeling hungry, stop eating, and burn the extra fat. It seems logical that obesity might be related to a deficiency of leptin. However, research has demonstrated that leptin levels are not always straightforward.

Contrary to what might be expected, obese individuals typically have high serum-leptin levels. Yet they also continue to have increased appetite and fat storage. The explanation:

Leptin resistance. Like insulin resistance, leptin resistance is characterized by high levels of leptin in the blood. Despite the surge in leptin from the increased fat production, its appetite-suppressing signal is not reaching the brain. When the brain cannot "hear" leptin, it thinks the body is "starving" and continues to send signals to increase appetite and fat storage. What blocks the leptin signal from reaching the brain? Chronic excess insulin.

Leptin Loses to Excess Insulin

Although leptin and insulin bind to separate receptors in the brain, they share a signaling cascade. In this shared cascade, excess insulin can (and does) block leptin signaling. There is a strong association between high levels of leptin, high levels of insulin, and insulin resistance in obese individuals. Without proper leptin signaling, appetite will be uncontrolled. Hunger signals will abound even when the body doesn't need more food, and this promotes overeating in an attempt to feel full and to fat storage due to faulty leptin signaling. This is not about willpower. It's about biochemistry.

Ready for Action: Cortisol

Cortisol is a hormone produced from cholesterol in the adrenal glands in response to exercise, waking up, and acute stress. Normally, cortisol has a predictable daily cycle that helps us wake up, exercise, and regulate energy properly. But it can also be called into action for acute stress. Cortisol allows us to "react" in a hurry for quick fight-or-flight decisions. Stress and cortisol go together. And when stress is high, cortisol is high.

In acute stress, cortisol will signal a flood of glucose (sugar) to be released for immediate use by large muscles needed for "fight or flight." Insulin is also temporarily inhibited by cortisol so that this glucose is not stored. Once a stress is relieved, cortisol will return to normal levels, and this acute cycle stops. Glucose does not continue to be released, and no increase in insulin will be required for this temporary situation. But stress is no longer temporary in our culture, and neither are cortisol responses. The fast-paced, sleep-deprived, high-sensory culture is perceived as unrelenting stress, and this leads to chronic elevated cortisol.

Why does this matter? Chronic elevated cortisol leads to insulin resistance (due to constantly elevated glucose) and causes fat to deposit in the abdomen. Chronically elevated cortisol has other significant effects in the body as well, but the main point is that insulin resistance is increased when cortisol remains elevated. Managing stress both physically and emotionally has a profound impact on our metabolism.

BLOOD SUGAR BLUES[12]

Sugar, or glucose, in the blood is an energy resource for your brain and muscles and general function. Our bodies prefer a limited range of blood sugar for maintaining energy and a sense of well-being. Ideally, fasting blood sugar (no food for 8 hours) is within 70–99 mg/dl. Normal blood sugar two hours after a meal is <140 mg/dl. The normal-functioning body will restore blood sugar to a range of 82–110 mg/dl.

What produces increases in blood sugar? We have only one hormone that will lower blood sugar, insulin, but multiple mechanisms in place to raise blood sugar. That's because excess blood sugar, until the introduction of the standard American diet, has not generally been the concern for our body. The concern was making sure the body would have enough energy stored in case of famine, since food supplies were not always predictable. Our body is most interested in making sure we have multiple ways to provide appropriate glucose in the blood. Several things can produce increases in blood sugar, including sugar production from the liver and the activity of certain hormones like cortisol, glucagon, growth hormone, and epinephrine.

However, food consumption is a big reason our blood sugar will rise, and this is where it gets interesting. Having a limited, slow rise in blood sugar is desirable for optimal cellular function, and this was commonly achieved in the diet prior to sugary, processed, and refined foods introduced into the modern diet. Now the body is exposed to large and rapid doses of easily available sugar from the processed and refined foods common in many diets, and this can upset this delicate system and eventually "break" it.

Excess blood sugar will be actively transported into cells by the hormone insulin to be stored as glycogen or fat. If this system breaks down and blood sugar isn't successfully transported or well regulated, remaining either too high or too low, it can cause life-threatening problems, including coma, kidney failure, and heart disease. Common problems associated with a lack of insulin or lack of insulin transport are high blood sugar >126 mg/dl (diabetes), abdominal weight gain, low energy, poor wound healing, heart disease, artherosclerosis, poor kidney function, neuropathy, confusion, seizures, blurred vision, and blindness.

Avoiding the "Panic of the Pancreas"

Generally, eating every four hours will help the body maintain appropriate blood sugar levels, preventing metabolic stress. Low blood-sugar levels can cause feelings of irritability or being "hangry." We need to be aware, however, that large doses of sugary or starchy refined foods can raise blood sugar very quickly and will be perceived as a crisis in the system. This "panic of the pancreas" will cause an overly large release of insulin to counteract the sudden surge in blood sugar, rapidly reducing it—too rapidly—resulting in an energy "crash" and the return of feelings of irritability and hunger. And so begins a cycle of metabolic stress.

Metabolic stress occurs when blood sugar is too low. Metabolic stress will trigger the hormones meant to raise your blood sugar. These are released, including cortisol and epinephrine. Epinephrine will make you nervous, but it will also stimulate your brain to crave carbohydrates. So you might eat a bowl of cereal or fruit and expect to have a minor increase in blood sugar, but your other stress hormones (including cortisol) will have signaled the muscles and the liver to produce and release glucose. Now your blood sugar is very high again, triggering another "panic of the pancreas," rapidly reducing blood sugar again. This is not ideal. It is a peak-and-valley energy crisis. This will eventually cause insulin resistance. This will also continually elevate your stress hormone, cortisol. The body prefers a slow, steady maintenance in blood sugar, over time, with moderate releases of insulin that will come from high-fiber carbohydrates and appropriate protein levels. This allows the body to feel satisfied and have reliable energy.

GLYCEMIC INDEX AND GLYCEMIC LOAD

Glycemic index and glycemic load are two related concepts. These tools try to quantify the impact that a food will have on your blood sugar and the subsequent release of insulin into the bloodstream. This is important for diabetics but also for everyone else, since rapid increases in blood sugar and insulin have serious metabolic consequences. This will be a very basic overview of the differences between glycemic index and glycemic load. These concepts are useful, but they are not without limitations.

The glycemic index reflects the amount of carbohydrates (sugar) in a specified quantity of food against the same quantity of table sugar (sucrose) and gives it a number. The glycemic index looks at four things: blood-sugar increase, insulin secretion, lipoprotein lipase (fat storage) stimulation, and the effect on the pancreas. The index also reflects the metabolic response to the percentages of fat, protein, and carbohydrate content of a food. The important thing to understand is this: If a food has a high glycemic index (>55), it has the potential to raise blood sugar quickly and cause a spike in insulin. Notice the word "potential." This is where the glycemic load becomes useful in the discussion.

Glycemic load is a function of the glycemic index but takes into account the total quantity of carbohydrates, as well as the quality, or amount of fiber, being consumed. And this changes everything. Suddenly carrots, which have a high glycemic index, become a low glycemic load choice due to their high fiber content. You would have to eat a lot of raw carrots to raise your blood sugar. This can also apply to candy. A small, single piece of candy, even though it is lacking in fiber, is not likely a large-enough quantity of carbohydrate to significantly raise blood sugar. Glycemic load is calculated as follows: GL = GI/100 × Net Carbs. Net carbs are equal to the total carbohydrates minus the dietary fiber. A low GL is <10. Above 20 is considered high.

Additionally, other factors can influence glycemic index and glycemic load. High-glycemic foods eaten in combination with other foods high in fiber and containing fat and protein can alter the overall metabolic response, generally reducing glycemic index (but this does not mean it is now low). Preparation methods also change glycemic response. If fiber is destroyed in cooking, the GI will go up. Temperature and pH of a food also change the glycemic response, with cold starches and acids slowing the blood-sugar increase. There are individual differences in glycemic response as well. Finally, the complexity of measuring GI and GL due to things like differences in ripeness of a food means that laboratories do not always arrive at the same result, causing unreliable data. Overreliance on the GI and GL for estimating blood sugar and insulin response in the real world will not provide enough certainty. GI and GL are simply *general* guides for understanding how a food might impact blood sugar and subsequent insulin response in the diet.

SECTION 3

TAKING THE JOURNEY
TO TRANSFORM YOUR
HEALTH—WHERE AM I, AND
HOW CAN I GET THERE?

CHAPTER 6

UNLOCKING THE SECRETS TO HEALTH TRANSFORMATION: USING FOOD TO YOUR ADVANTAGE

FOOD IS NOT THE ENEMY—IGNORANCE IS!

WE NEED TO KNOW IF WE'RE helping or hurting our body. Are we moving toward health or toward disease? One way to understand this is to record what we eat. In a normal individual, recording food intake is a great way to learn about our nutritional status—are you lacking vitamins and minerals? Do you need more protein? It helps us to know where our diet might need adjustment.

Real Life:

THE SALTY NURSING STUDENT and THE COST OF BINGE DRINKING

Every semester, my nursing students were required to record their food intake over a three-day period. These records were collected, coded to protect identity, and redistributed to a fellow "nurse" in the class for further evaluation and recommendations. There was one rule for recommendations: No vitamin supplements, except vitamin D, were allowed to be used to compensate for nutritional deficiencies. This was a big academic assignment, worth big points. It was explained that the focus of grading was not on the quality of the dietary intake but on the evaluation of the intake and subsequent nutritional recommendations. The primary goal was to have students make a personal connection between food intake, nutritional status, and long-term health outcomes. Through the use of personal dietary intakes, this "real life" experience created an opportunity to transform the way these future nurses understood and applied nutritional knowledge to themselves and their patients. It was meant to teach them the difficulty of evaluating someone's most personal choice—their diet—and help them engage in becoming health facilitators, not nutritional dictators.

The students were often surprised by how emotional and informative this assignment was. When students actually reviewed the details of their dietary intake and understood the impact on current and future health, it had a tendency to evoke strong feelings. As an educator, I generally witnessed one of three emotions after students understood their dietary intake: 1) anger or distress; 2) excitement, or 3) sadness. Why? Well, we're often comfortably ignorant about the details of our dietary intake. People like to feel that their diet is "healthy" without ever actually recording intake. The angry students were quite shocked by the deficiencies in their diet, and many felt betrayed by their favorite foods, often promoted as "healthy" but loaded with sodium and sugar and lacking nutrients. The excited students, although also nutritionally challenged in many cases, felt empowered by the information. The sad students were often discouraged by the awareness that a dietary shift was needed in order to better address nutritional needs; they felt overwhelmed and fearful that they wouldn't be able to "enjoy" their new diet. All the students described how difficult it was to diplomatically offer recommendations and invitations for change when they assumed the role of "nurse." This is not unlike working with a patient!

A couple of student experiences stand out as interesting for their insight into how dietary analysis can impact knowledge and inspire personal change, and I would like to share these with you. The first student had diligently completed his three-day intake and learned, to his dismay, that his daily sodium intake averaged more than 10,000 mg per day. That is more than three times the recommended upper-limit intake of 2,300 mg/day for sodium! (One teaspoon of table salt contains more than 2,300 mg of sodium.) This student was visibly upset as he explained that he just couldn't understand how that was possible until he closely examined his intake of processed meats, i.e., deli meats and some other convenience foods. And then he began to understand the risks he was taking with this diet. He became fully aware of the link between sodium intake and increased blood pressure. He mentioned that his father had suffered a heart attack and was concerned for his own future heart health. He was clearly reassessing his diet.

The semester ended, and I didn't see this student for a couple of semesters, until one day when he approached me in the hallway and excitedly exclaimed how he had changed his diet after the nutrition course. He reported that he had experienced improved blood pressure and weight distribution, and didn't feel "hungry" or deprived. Instead, he felt better generally and had more energy. The nutritional knowledge he had gained in the course was being practiced in his daily living and, according to him, had "changed his life." Can you imagine the impact this nurse will have when interacting with patients about lifestyle and dietary choices?

The second student was notable in that she clearly did not attempt to hide anything about her dietary intake, which proved very interesting. She definitely trusted that the grade for this assignment would be based on the analysis and recommendations, not the intake. She told it like it was! After we collected her three-day dietary record, it was noted that intake for one evening had included significant alcohol consumption. Apparently this student had been "binge" drinking at a party and had bravely recorded it on her intake. It was also clear that her food consumption during that evening and the following day was rather limited. She had basically had only one day out of three that was a more "typical" food-intake day with several meals. (Her intake was subsequently analyzed by a fellow student "nurse" and was, in my opinion, one of the more difficult "patients" to make recommendations for—where do you start, and how do you say it?)

After taking an opportunity to speak with the student privately, I reaffirmed her courage in completing the assignment with her actual intake, praised her for her honesty, and thanked her for being willing to explore her dietary intake in a very real way. And she did explore it. She was shocked when she understood the full impact that the binge drinking had on not only her caloric intake but also her nutrient intake. She was rather surprised at the number of calories quickly consumed in one evening and the resulting negligible nutrient intake. The subsequent "hangover" then impacted her nutrient intake the following day, resulting in almost no food intake early in the day and poor food intake into the evening. This student began to internalize the reality that the body needs nutrients all day, every day, and that it's challenging enough without inviting loads of empty calories and toxins that need to be dealt with in the liver. She recognized that this behavior seriously compromised her nutrition in so many ways, and she expressed that she was rethinking her nutritional choices and self-care behaviors.

Wow! Again, we did not grade the students on whether they changed their diet or followed the recommendations. Any change a student undertook after this assignment remained a strictly personal decision. Of course, it was hoped that optimal dietary intakes might be considered and applied, but at least every student became aware of their actual intake and knew the potential health impact. More importantly, I hold onto the hope that these personal nutrition experiences will someday positively influence patient care.

A CALL TO ACTION: KNOWING WHAT'S REALLY, ACTUALLY, TRUTHFULLY IN YOUR DIET

Dietary Analysis

The quickest and easiest way to learn about our diet is to keep a food diary for three consecutive days, with one day being a weekend day. This three-day diary will give a general idea of your food choices, how much protein, fat, and carbohydrates you are consuming, and whether something like Vitamin A status is in the optimal range. If someone is really ambitious, a two-week diary can be kept. (Two weeks is considered more accurate and reliable for predicting long-term health status, but it is, obviously, more time consuming.)

Tools for this task:

Measuring cups, spoons, and, if possible, a food scale for measuring portion sizes. (Yes, you need to measure if you want to be accurate!)

Dietary Intake Diary or Notebook

A notebook used to record all of the food eaten in each 24-hour period, including amounts or portions. You must also record beverages. This method will require you to look up information on each food from a reliable resource (including the food label) to record nutrient content, calculate total calories, establish nutrient content for each vitamin in a food, fiber content, sugar content, and the ratio of fats, carbohydrates, and protein (this ratio will add up to 100%) that are consumed that day.

Or you can use an app, such as My Fitness Pal, that will automatically compute this information once you enter the food and the amount eaten. Food can also be entered automatically using the bar code feature on the app. Additionally, macronutrient ratios can be adjusted to reflect your consumption goals. Acquire an app on your smartphone or similar program on the computer. Basic apps or computer programs are free, and these are sufficient for the purpose of recording food intake. Be prepared to enter some basic information (height, weight, gender, exercise or activity level). Once you have completed your dietary intake record, nutritional reports from the app can be generated. The following information should be provided by the app:

> Intake/Status of Nutrients: Vitamin A, Vitamin C, Calcium, Iron, Sodium, Potassium—some apps will give a more extensive intake record, perhaps including magnesium, zinc, etc., which can be even more helpful.

> Fiber Intake

> Sugar Intake

> Calorie Intake

> Macronutrients (Fat, Carbs, Protein) Ratios

Paper to record items not recorded by an app:

> Record water intake (tracking hydration)

> Take the opportunity to record your sleep habits during this time.

Here are examples of a breakfast entry:

3 large eggs
1 slice pork bacon
1 slice of 100% whole-grain toast
1 teaspoon butter
½ grapefruit

Or

1 cup steel-cut oats
½ cup fresh blueberries
½ cup Greek yogurt
1 tsp raw honey
1 tsp cinnamon

Be specific about the food you eat, for example, record "steel-cut oats" instead of just recording "oatmeal." Also try to record your intake as soon after the meal as you can. Recording your diet in the evening by using recall is not as accurate. You may forget to add the afternoon snack or under- or overestimate the amount you ate. Sometimes, if you wait too long, you won't be able to recall the meal accurately enough to create useful data. It is only three days, so commit to measuring portions BEFORE you begin eating, and begin recording as you consume the meal or shortly afterward.

Once you have recorded three days of food intake and generated reports, you should be able to gain a basic understanding of your nutritional intake, including potential trouble spots that need more attention in the diet. This data can also provide inspiration for making helpful food choices in the future. Maybe you need to get more magnesium or calcium. Maybe your sodium is extremely high. Maybe you need more fiber. Your protein intake might be on target, but your carbohydrates and fats might need some adjusting. This is where you can access the internet to learn about foods that might be helpful for increasing a nutrient or about tips for reducing sodium intake. Or you can learn about good fiber sources and start adding these foods into the diet.

CAUTION: "health apps" or "programs" will often focus on calorie counting and weight loss. This is NOT a focus that will provide long-term health and maintain optimal weight. Some will also provide social media groups as well as their own "helpful tips" about your caloric intake, exercise level, and macronutrient ratios, but much of the advice is not scientifically sound. Be especially cautious about free advice given from self-proclaimed "nutrition experts/journalists" in any social media forum or magazine. Unless the individuals have professional nutrition or related scientific credentials from an accredited university, they are not qualified to fully evaluate the usefulness or health impact of a particular diet.

THE ANSWERS IN YOUR BLOOD: WORKING WITH YOUR DOCTOR

Another option for understanding your health and nutritional status is to obtain blood work from a qualified lab. You can have your doctor order blood tests, or you can contract with a laboratory online or locally. Some online tests can be ordered and done at home using a finger stick, or you can go to a local blood-draw center. Insurance will often provide coverage for blood tests when ordered by your doctor but will not cover tests without a doctor's order. Ask questions about what tests are covered by your insurance. Be aware that blood work will incur costs versus a dietary analysis but can provide a lot more detail about certain nutrients. Blood work can also provide specific data about certain organ or gland function that cannot be determined by dietary records.

Here are some possible blood tests:

Vitamin D:

Even though we can obtain 90% of our vitamin D through 15–20 minutes of daily sun exposure on our skin, many people, even in sunny climates, are low in this vitamin due to stress and excessive use of sunscreen. This vitamin (which actually becomes a hormone) has many roles but is especially important for thyroid health, immune function, healthy blood pressure, increasing absorption of calcium and phosphorous, healthy skin, bones, teeth, and mood. A blood level as low as 20 ng/ml can be adequate for some individuals, but it is not considered optimal. Serum levels of 30 ng/ml are considered the minimum target for receiving a significant benefit from vitamin D.[13] Optimal levels are anywhere from 40 to 80 ng/ml. A range of 50 to 60 ng/ml is a good target.[14] Levels which exceed 80 ng/ml can cause serious side effects, including pancreatitis.

If vitamin D is low, a D_3 supplement between 2,000 IU and 5,000 IU is generally recommended, but 10,0000 IU may be useful in severe deficiencies. Once adequate blood levels are present, a supplement of 5,000 IU or less is generally sufficient and recommended, since vitamin D it is not readily available from food and not reliably obtained in the diet. The only way to know your vitamin D status is to take a blood test, known as Vitamin D 25(OH)D.

Liver Function:

The liver is the body's detox center for the blood. It processes medications, nutrients, and hormones, and produces clotting factors. It also stores bile, fat, cholesterol, and vitamins, and can produce glucose. The liver is a very busy organ that is subject to damage from toxic medications, alcohol, dietary factors, and physical injury. Normally, the liver enzymes are contained only within the liver cells, but these enzymes will spill into the bloodstream when the liver is stressed or injured. Elevated liver enzymes in the blood can indicate celiac disease, insulin resistance, and liver diseases like fatty liver, which have dietary origins related to carbohydrate and sugar intake. Liver damage rarely presents with obvious symptoms until it is advanced and life threatening, so monitoring liver enzymes can provide insight into how your liver is functioning long before a more serious problem develops. In a liver enzyme test, two main enzymes are tested: ALT (alanine aminotransferase) and AST (aspartate aminotransferase).

Hemoglobin A1C:

This test measures your average blood sugar occurring over a six-week period and is not influenced by sudden daily fluctuations in diet. It's the long-term view of your blood-sugar health. In general, hemoglobin A1C creates inflammation and stress in the body and is a marker for diabetes. Elevated A1C accelerates aging and promotes inflammatory conditions like heart disease and dementia. When this number is more than 6, the patient is considered diabetic. Ideally, this should be less than 5.5.

Fasting Glucose:
This test is done after a period of fasting at least eight hours, without food or liquid (other than water). It is done to diagnose both type 1 and type 2 diabetes. This is often the only glucose test offered to patients and, while valuable, is inadequate for accurately diagnosing all diabetics, since it cannot identify those who are insulin resistant already and progressing to type 2 diabetes. Fasting blood sugar should be below 100 mg/dL.

Insulin Response Test and Glucose Tolerance Test:
This test measures glucose and insulin after fasting and two hours after a 75 gm glucose drink. Insulin resistance is not exclusive to obese patients, so it is important to have this test regardless of your weight. It is well known that blood sugar can remain in the normal range for ten to twenty years while excess insulin compensates for resistance to insulin. Relying on glucose alone can give misleading health information about how your body is handling sugar. By measuring insulin levels in addition to glucose, insulin resistance can be detected many years before type 2 diabetes fully develops.

This information can be useful in helping a patient with high insulin values consider important dietary changes which can halt progression of insulin resistance and prevent development of type 2 diabetes in the first place.

Normal value for glucose tolerance at two hours following the drink is 140 mg/dL. Normal fasting insulin should be less than 10 and ideally 6; values above 10 automatically indicate insulin resistance. Insulin level two hours after the drink should be less than 50. Insulin levels between 60 and 100 after two hours is considered borderline insulin resistant, and levels of more than 100 are considered resistant. If all insulin values remain below 30, pancreatic exhaustion is likely, due to many years of high insulin output; this is an inadequate insulin response and will generally be accompanied by high glucose values in the diabetic range.

High-Sensitivity C-Reactive Protein (CRP):
The high-sensitivity CRP test measures chronic inflammation which is specific to the blood vessels. Since artherosclerosis is an inflammatory disease, this test can be useful for understanding your risk for inflammatory processes like artherosclerosis and heart disease (CVD). A high-sensitivity CRP less than 1 mg/L is ideal. A CRP of more than 3 mg/L indicates more serious inflammation is occurring and correlates with elevated HA1C and increased risk of type 2 diabetes. This test is not useful as an indicator of cardiovascular risk if an autoimmune disease is already present, since inflammation will be widespread in the body, with CRP levels much higher than 3 mg/L.

Thyroid Function Panel:

The comprehensive thyroid panel includes the following tests:

1. TSH (thyroid stimulating hormone)
2. T_4 (free thyroxine)
3. T_3 (total AND free T_3)
4. Antibody test: TPO and Tg; or TSHRAb (specific to Grave's)
5. Consider a thyroid ultrasound

It is important to test more than just TSH to determine real thyroid function and whether there is an autoimmune disease affecting the thyroid. When thyroid function is low, it's known as hypothyroidism. Symptoms of low thyroid include fatigue, depression, anxiety, dry skin and hair, thinning hair, excessive weight gain, constipation, carpel tunnel, infertility/miscarriage, and sensitivity to cold temperatures. Hyperthyroidism, or Grave's disease, indicates an overactive thyroid, and this can cause the eyes to protrude from the face, increase heat sensitivity, increase appetite, cause rapid, unexplained weight loss, hand tremors, insomnia, loss of endurance, anxiety, and difficulty concentrating. If a high level of TPO antibody is occurring, an autoimmune disease, Hashimoto thyroiditis, is present (although this is not the only way to diagnose Hashimoto's). Hashimoto's correlates strongly with the presence of hypothyroidism and is present in up to 95% of patients with hypothyroidism.

The tricky part about thyroid tests is in the interpretation. Guidelines from the National Academy of Clinical Biochemists recommend a range of TSH between 1.0 and 4.5 mIU/L as normal. However, it is indicated that this range will likely be reduced to 1.0 and 2.5 mIU/L in the future, based on long-term studies of patients. With all this variation, it's important to remember to treat the patient and not just the lab result, because some patients will feel strongly symptomatic with a TSH at a 3 and respond well to treatment for hypothyroidism. So if a TSH is "normal" and a patient symptomatic, it is not unreasonable to consider that hypothyroidism may still be a factor. In these cases, you need to be asking a lot of questions and looking closely at the other thyroid tests, since TSH can be normal while T_3 is low, indicating a problem, and TPO antibodies may be high—also a problem. A TSH <0.5 mIU/L can indicate hyperthyroidism, or Grave's disease. It is important to state that the TSH during pregnancy will fluctuate and has a separate and specific recommended range.

Most commonly, a patient with hypothyroidism will receive a prescription for T_4 only, a form of thyroid hormone that requires conversion by the body to the active form, T_3, and this works for many patients. However, some patients remain symptomatic and struggle to feel well. It is important to know that a combination treatment of T_4 and T_3 might be considered in these cases, especially since some individuals have a genetic issue that affects conversion of T_4. When symptoms remain and TSH is "normal" and T_3 is in the mid-range of "normal," it is important to consider that a patient might need more interventions, such as additional T_3 over and above what is offered in the combination prescription.

These patients may need to bring T_3 levels as high as upper quartile of "normal" to resolve symptoms. This is very much a "Goldilocks" pursuit—the treatment needs to be "just right" for each patient. Again, never rely on one test when evaluating thyroid function.

Autoimmunity Is a Separate Issue

When autoimmunity, like Hashimoto's, is present, it is crucial to address it in addition to hypo- or hyperthyroidism. Thyroid medication does not address Hashimoto's thyroiditis. Hashimoto's thyroiditis is a separate issue from the hyper- or hypothyroidism and needs treatment specific to autoimmunity. In general, autoimmunity indicates that the body is attacking itself, and inflammation will be present. In the case of Hashimoto's, inflammation is manifesting in the thyroid.

The gut (digestive tract) is also compromised in cases of autoimmunity, and food allergies and sensitivities should be identified and addressed. An overgrowth of bacteria in the small intestine, parasites, fungal infections, and yeast overgrowth (*Candida albicans*) may also contribute to gut issues and contribute to the autoimmunity. When the gut is compromised and inflamed, nutrient malabsorption is of concern. It is important to consider nutritional deficiencies, especially selenium, in these cases. Supplemental iodine, which may be necessary in iodine-deficient cases of hypothyroidism, is not initially advised in someone with Hashimoto's until the inflammation of autoimmunity can be addressed.

NMR Lipid Profile:

This gives information about triglycerides, total cholesterol, HDL (good cholesterol) and LDL cholesterol, but it also gives you the NUMBER of LDL-P (lipoprotein particles: these particles carry the cholesterol around in your vessels like a passenger in a car). The number of particles is a much better predictor for heart attack risk than just knowing LDL cholesterol, because it's the particles that attach to the vessel walls that cause damage. The more particles there are, the greater the opportunity for damage to occur. Triglycerides should be less than 150 mg/dL and, ideally, less than 100 mg/dL. LDL should be less than 100 mg/dL for both men and women. HDL should be more than 40 mg/dL for men and 60 mg/dL for women. While total cholesterol less than 200 mg/dL is considered desirable, the total number is less important than the overall profile that includes the ratio of cholesterol to HDL. The ratio of HDL to total cholesterol should be less than 3.5:1 for a lower-than-average risk of heart disease. For instance, if total cholesterol is more than 300 but HDL is 100, this is less concerning than a total cholesterol of 150 and an HDL of 30. Triglyceride to HDL ratio is ideally 1:1, but 2:1 is acceptable. When HDL is less than 60 and triglycerides are more than 100, insulin resistance might be happening. An HDL of less than 40 with triglycerides of more than 150 can indicate diabetes and a buildup of plaque in the arteries, increasing the risk of coronary disease. It isn't about total cholesterol—it's about ratios, triglycerides, and LDL-P numbers.

Testosterone for Men Over Forty:
Testosterone begins to decline gradually after thirty-five years of age, and levels should be checked due to an increased risk of developing type 2 diabetes when testosterone remains too low over a period of time. Low testosterone can contribute to increasing abdominal fat and waist circumference (hence the risk of type 2 diabetes), as well as muscle loss and weakness, tiredness, foggy thinking, and mood swings. There is an optimal zone for testosterone, and blood levels must be carefully monitored by a physician.

THE GENES YOU WEAR

Are genetics destiny? No. Genes provide a blueprint of possibilities within us, but we do not express every gene during our lifetime. Gene expression is affected by several external factors, including age, environment, and lifestyle/nutrition. This impact of external influences on gene expression is known as epigenetics and is providing important understanding about how we might influence gene expression by lifestyle and nutrition choices. What we choose to eat and how we choose to live can have significant impact on how our genes ultimately express and affect our health.

By understanding our genetic profile, we can be aware of the genes we carry that influence the risk of certain types of disease, cancer, or obesity. This knowledge can help us be more intentional about our habits and lifestyle, potentially avoiding certain dietary intakes that might aggravate a condition. It can feel overwhelming to have so much information, but it can also be empowering to know what might help or hinder your genetic expression. It can be as simple as knowing that you should avoid high intakes of saturated fat in the diet in favor of unsaturated fats because you don't metabolize that type of fat as well as another genotype. It might inform you that you are highly sensitive to caffeine or are unable to metabolize alcohol. It might also reveal that you are lacking certain enzymes that process vitamins due to a recessive gene and need to supplement with specialized forms of folate (L-methylfolate, NOT folic acid) and B-12 in the form of methylcobalamin (NOT cyanocobalamin) to protect against immune disorders, depression, or neural-tube birth defects.

How do you know what genetic information is in you? You get a DNA test. DNA tests are much more accessible than ever before, can be ordered online, and don't require a blood test, just saliva. Once the results are obtained, further evaluation of the information is necessary, but these can be done online in minutes for a small fee.

CHAPTER 7

COMMIT! TO FEEDING YOURSELF WITH PURPOSE

SO HOW DO I FEED MYSELF?

THE ANSWER IS SIMPLE: Eat Food. With intention. Not food-like products. The grocery store carries both, but don't be fooled. And limit sugar, especially added sugar.

Eat REAL, WHOLE FOODS. You can identify a whole food by its simplicity. Missing is the fancy packaging and long ingredient lists full of unrecognizable words on the label. Real food generally resembles what is found in nature, rarely contains more than a few ingredients, and is DELICIOUS when properly prepared. Real food is not made in a chemistry lab, composed of ingredients that may be used in industrial manufacturing, or possess colors that belong only in a paint store.

EXAMPLES OF REAL FOOD:

Real, whole foods include wild or grass-fed meats and wild-caught seafood, pasture-raised chicken and eggs, fresh vegetables and fruits, beans, lentils, raw nuts, seeds, and whole grains. Avocados, olives, cold-pressed, extra-virgin olive oil, cold-pressed, unrefined coconut oil, and grass-fed butter are all excellent dietary choices. Frozen vegetables are options when fresh are unavailable. Canned beans like pinto, black, or kidney are also a good option but should not include any sauces (you can make your own low-sugar sauces) or additives like sugar. Canned tomatoes and tomato sauces with no added sugar are also good choices, but otherwise avoid other canned fruits and vegetables, since they have few nutrients and little or no fiber left in them.

Fresh vegetables and fruits are available year round and are important to consume regularly. It is not necessary to cook or peel the majority of your fruits and vegetables, but it is a good idea to wash them in plenty of clean water before consuming. In fact, many fruits and vegetables are the ultimate convenience food, since they come prepackaged and ready to eat—carrots, radishes, peppers, apples, bananas, and oranges. The only difference for these convenience foods is that they don't have a lengthy shelf life and need to be eaten within a few days. Many greens now come packaged in ready-to-eat containers—just beware of the dressings and other add-ins that may also be offered. (Make your own full-fat dressings, and avoid vegetable oils like corn, peanut, safflower, canola, and soybean. This will be discussed later in the book.)

Meats from wild and pasture-raised sources are important to understand for their protein and fat content. The protein available in animal foods is praised for its content of all necessary amino acids, and this is appropriate. The saturated fat content of pasture-raised and wild animals has been criticized, however, and this is not appropriate. Saturated and other fats from pasture-raised and wild meat sources can make important contributions to our health, including raising the "good" HDL cholesterol, and are not associated with increased risk of heart disease. Thankfully, current data, both clinical and epidemiological, is overcoming the incorrect assumption that consuming saturated fat is the cause of heart disease.

In contrast to wild and pasture-raised meats, conventionally raised beef and poultry will not contain the same fat ratio of omega-6 to omega-3. Pasture-raised or wild meats contain higher amounts of omega-3 fats, which are anti-inflammatory, and lower saturated fat overall vs. conventionally raised grain-fed livestock, which contains a much higher amount of pro-inflammatory omega-6 fats. Cows are meant to eat grass, not grain, yet grain is the predominant food for livestock in the United States, and it has changed the nature of the meat, most notably increasing the ratio of omega-6 to omega-3s in the fat of the animal. Conventionally raised meat contains more pro-inflammatory fat.

Conventionally raised cattle are also given hormones and antibiotics to promote growth and prevent or treat the infections commonly seen in large feed lots. The fat and muscle of this livestock will contain antibiotic and hormone residues, along with potentially more pesticide residues from the grain in the diet. Conventionally raised poultry are given medications as well as antibiotics in their feed and water, but this varies between producers, and the term "no antibiotics ever" still remains controversial in how exposure is defined. Conventionally raised poultry, unlike cattle, will not receive steroids or hormones since this practice has been banned for more than fifty years by federal law, so this is not a distinction on the label that matters.

The distinction between grass-fed and wild vs. grain-fed (corn or soy) meats also applies to the products produced from these animals. The fat of butter from a grass-fed cow is different from that of a grain-fed cow. Cheese, milk, yogurt, and eggs will also have differences in their fat based on how the animal was fed. "Cage-free" status is not the same as "free-range"; "free range" is not the same as "pasture raised"; the term "organic" does NOT refer to being grass fed, pasture raised, or wild.

Eat a variety of foods
Do not rely on supplements to repair a deficient diet.

COOKED OR RAW?
Should I cook it? Can I eat it raw? Both cooked and raw foods have their merits when it comes to supporting optimal nutrition. Some minerals are more available when food is cooked; some vitamins are more abundant when food remains raw. Eating at least half of the diet in a raw and minimally processed state ensures access to fiber and vitamins and enzymes that are sensitive to heat. ("Raw" describes a food that is not heated above 118° F at any time during preparation.) Not all cooking methods will enhance availability of nutrients.

Fortunately, cooking methods that promote availability of nutrients are not complicated.

Raw and minimally processed foods can include low heating, sprouting, and dehydrating. All fresh produce is raw. Pasteurized foods are not raw. Nuts and seeds are raw if the label states that they are raw; otherwise, assume they are roasted or pasteurized. Nuts, seeds, grains, and legumes may be sprouted and are still considered raw. Sprouting can enhance vitamin content and digestibility of a food by reducing lectins, which block nutrient absorption (sprouted raw kidney beans and alfalfa sprouts still have high lectin content and should not be consumed).

Other raw foods include rolled grains and fruits and vegetables in their natural or fermented state. Fermented foods that are not heat processed are described as "live" and include sauerkraut, kimchi, raw pickles, kombucha, yogurt, and kefir as rich sources of probiotics. Live fermented foods can help improve gut health. Rolled oats or other rolled grains are considered raw since they are only minimally processed by pressing or "rolling" and still contain many enzymes, heat-sensitive vitamins, and fiber. However, many commercial rolled grains are also steam treated and are no longer considered raw but still remain a highly nutritious, minimally processed option. Rolled grains do not need to be cooked to be eaten. Instant oatmeal is highly processed and should be avoided. Ground flour, even whole grain, does not fall into the category of raw or unprocessed since the fiber is significantly destroyed by grinding, and it should not be a dietary staple.

(Ground grain flour, even when it's from the whole-grain kernel, behaves like a simple sugar in the bloodstream.)

Eating a salad with a healthy full-fat dressing is an excellent nutritional choice. The vitamins A, D, E, and K found in green leafy vegetables, and other produce actually require fat to be absorbed, so salad dressing is a critical component to a healthy salad. Learning to make healthy fat-based salad dressings requires only basic kitchen skills and equipment and quickly creates a nutritious and delicious food.

When it comes to cooking food, the idea is to maintain as much flavor and nutrition as possible. Helpful cooking methods include low heating, baking or roasting, steaming, simmering, and sautéing. Steaming and lightly sautéing can help enhance availability of nutrients such as calcium in vegetables like broccoli and kale. Other preparation methods include soaking prior to cooking. Dry beans, grains, and nuts can benefit from extended soaking (24 hours) to help remove or reduce the nutrient-blocking lectins and phytates prior to cooking. Cooking whole grains after soaking is really fast and makes for wonderful cereals...no grinding needed. Steaming is superior to boiling for retaining nutrients.

Slow cookers are a wonderful addition to any healthy kitchen. Even pressure cookers can have their place when it comes to cooking soaked beans, although not a necessary kitchen item. Slow cookers make delicious and healthy broths and soups, as well as excellent tenderizers for tougher cuts of meat. A well-made broth in a slow cooker can provide extra nutritional support to the gut and help with joint pain. Slow cookers are also great for cooking whole-grain cereals (while you sleep) or beans.

WHAT ABOUT SUGAR?

According to the USDA Average Daily Intake Data by Food Source, from 2007–2010, Americans consumed an average of 17.73 teaspoons a day from added sugar. Adults consumed 17.50 teaspoons, while children consumed 18.43 teaspoons! Surprisingly, fast food accounted for only about 1.6 teaspoons per day of this added sugar. More shocking was the data that estimated 13 teaspoons per day were being consumed at home. So it isn't just about blaming fast food for adding sugar to the diet. It's about the refined and processed foods and juices eaten at home. Eighteen teaspoons per day is a lot of sugar, and it has effects on our cardiovascular health, according to the American Heart Association. In fact, the impact is significant enough that official recommendations on sugar were published by the American Heart Association in 2009, due to concerns about America's increasing sugar consumption.

What are the recommendations for sugar?

The American Heart Association (AHA) recommended in 2009 that added sugar consumption be limited to six teaspoons per day for adult women and nine teaspoons per day for adult males. In 2016, the AHA included children in its official scientific statement and recommended **no added sugar for children younger than two** and a six-teaspoon-per-day limit on children older than two.

How do you measure sugar?

Each teaspoon of sugar is equal to 4 grams, so, according to the AHA, women and children older than two should not exceed 24 grams/day of added sugar, and men, 36 grams/day. This is a *limit*, not a *goal!* As a nutritionist, I think it is a good idea to account for all of the grams of sugar being consumed in a day, especially for children, since sugar consumption, in general, can be deceptively easy. For example, 100% fruit juices might not be considered sweetened with "added" sugar, but they are a naturally occurring simple-sugar source, lack fiber, and significantly contribute to overall sugar consumption. If fruit is eaten in its whole state, raw (so it includes the fiber), it is not a significant source of sugar for the average healthy individual.

BEWARE OF THE MANY NAMES FOR SUGAR

It would be easy to account for added sugar in the diet if it appeared by only a few names, like sucrose, cane sugar, high-fructose corn syrup, corn syrup, or fructose, but there are more than fifty-six different names (and counting!) for sugar that can legally appear on a food label in America. Why so many names? By law, an ingredient gets listed by volume on the label. The highest-volume ingredient gets listed first. By having multiple names for sweeteners in a food product, they are no longer compiled under the umbrella of "sugar" and can appear as a separate and less-voluminous ingredient. Separately listing the different sugars is an easy way to make sugar "disappear" down the list in an unrecognizable form. If these sweeteners were all listed as the added sugar they are, sugar would be the first ingredient on many food-product labels!

One way to combat this problem with the ingredient list is to look at the Nutrition Facts food label under the carbohydrate section. The label will list the total sugars; however, this will not separate naturally occurring sugars and the added sugars. The next step is to try to find a similar product that claims no added sugar and compare the difference between the sugar content. This is a limited way to account for added sugars and works only when you can compare a similar food that claims "no added sugar" on the label. It serves as reference point as to how much sugar is actually added. There is no current legal requirement to separate the added sugars from the naturally occurring sugars on the Nutrition Facts label.

Sugar consumption, especially with diabetics, is a concern because of its ability to immediately raise blood-sugar and effect insulin needs. However, there is one type of commonly used sugar, fructose, that won't immediately raise blood sugar, and this can create a false sense of protection for a diabetic or anyone concerned about their health. Fructose doesn't need to raise blood sugar to trigger excess insulin release or initiate fat storage in the liver; it happens indirectly and can create a fatty liver. It is a cautionary tale about how differently certain sugars can operate when it comes to fat storage in the liver and promoting excess insulin production. It isn't just about blood sugar. Reviewing this is important when making sweetener choices, because fructose is used not only as a concentrated ingredient to sweeten products, but it is also the sugar molecule of agave syrup. All sugars have metabolic consequences.

BEWARE OF FAKE FOOD

This may sound a bit silly, but many Americans consume large amounts of items that aren't actually food, in the nutritional sense. Fake food can be found in restaurants, schools, sport clubs, and even hospitals. A convenient, pre-packaged item may "look" like food, but it has been largely stripped of its nutritional richness through processing. It may include pictures of whole foods like fruits on the packaging, but the ingredient label will expose that the item does not actually contain the fruit or its juice; it's just filled with flavorings and sugars. Additional ingredients are often added to enhance color, texture, extend the shelf life (preserve), and supercharge the flavor so you'll buy more. These extra ingredients can be harmful in ways you might not expect, affecting hormones and appetite.[15] These products are legal, but they aren't legitimate as nutritious and health-promoting foods.

Evidence? Products with beautiful pictures of fresh blueberries on the packaging or the word "blueberry" written on the label may not contain blueberries at all.[16, 17] For example, Quaker brand multigrain crisps prominently feature the words "wild blueberry" while minimizing the word "flavor." Furthermore, the blueberry "flavor" remains a mystery altogether since there isn't even a mention of actual blueberries—or their juice—in the ingredient list. Kellogg's blueberry frosted mini-wheats also contain no blueberries, despite the depiction of the animated mini-wheat juggling fresh berries on the package. The frosting is just sugars, flavorings, and coloring. Examples of products with no actual blueberries but only fake blueberry-like bits include Hungry

Jack Complete Blueberry Wheat Pancake and Waffle Mix, Betty Crocker Blueberry Muffin Mix, Jiffy Blueberry Muffin Mix, and blueberry bagels sold at Target. Yoplait blueberry pie yogurt contains no blueberries but derives blueberry flavor from sugars, artificial flavorings, and food coloring. Blueberry Craisins do not contain whole blueberries, but are cranberries infused with blueberry concentrate, which is listed as a fourth ingredient on the label.

Let's talk about the prepared "lunches" for children that come in attractive, shelf-stable packaging. Besides often containing the fake-fruit products mentioned above, they also contain objectionable ingredients in the "meats" and crackers.[18] The 100% turkey label on one lunch product might lead you to believe that this is simply sliced turkey, but this turkey also contains water, potassium lactate, modified corn starch, salt, dextrose, carrageenan, sodium phosphates, sodium diacetate, sodium ascorbate, sodium nitrite, natural and artificial flavor, and smoke flavor. What's 100% about that turkey meat? Even more alarming is that partially hydrogenated oil, a dangerous "trans-fat" that will be discussed later in the book, is still found in the ingredient list of some of the lunch offerings. Not surprisingly, these convenient lunch options, marketed to busy parents and nutritionally deprived youngsters, also contain close to the USDA-recommended sodium for the entire day. Interestingly, there is a website with the word "parent" in its address that is devoted to displaying the "nutritional highlights" of these lunch packs but is nothing more than a marketing site sponsored by the manufacturer.[19] Remember, nutrition is not the goal for the manufacturer—just convenience, shelf life, and enticing flavors meant to promote repeat purchases.

The Fake Food Mindset: A Social Disconnect

The other more subtle downside surrounding fake food is the instant-gratification factor promoted by a no-preparation format. It creates the illusion that cooking and food preparation shouldn't intrude on our precious time and that this "problem" of having to dice an apple, assemble a sandwich, and make a meal is "solved" by outsourcing our diets to industry. "Meals" will be provided in the format of the manufacturer's choosing. The message is that you do not need to spend time considering what you eat—just grab and go! You should not have to bother about the details of your food intake. Your busy life should remain the priority. In this environment, planning and choosing food for well-balanced meals eventually becomes a mystery, since it is not practiced in any real way. And this has deeper impact.

What originally felt like a food choice is no longer a choice, because you no longer learn or maintain the skills needed to plan for, shop for, and prepare healthy and economical meals. This creates a disconnection from our food, and mindless eating emerges, creating a void physically and emotionally. Opportunities for enhanced nutrition and the expression of choice and creativity in our diet are diminished. Connection with our food producers and the positive social interaction that occurs when people cook together disappears. The enhanced self-care that comes from these experiences is lost.

When food manufacturers decide your intake, your skill set for self-care and positive social connection surrounding food is disrupted. Does this sound like a recipe for optimal health? (To be clear, convenience is not always a negative choice, but it is important to be mindful of how and what we consume for "convenience.")

BEWARE OF THE HEALTH HALO

Some foods are promoted as healthy, and everything about the way they look seems to portray a healthy content; but, in reality, they are not healthy, and hence the "health halo." This "health halo" phenomenon relies on the impression that a product is healthier than it actually is because the label contains words like "whole wheat," "organic," "real fruit," "fat free," "yogurt," "protein," or "100% natural." The label may also claim it has a full day's supply of a certain vitamin or fiber or is heart healthy or is low in cholesterol, but don't believe the hype that this food is somehow healthy. Many of these nutritional "buzz" words are not clearly defined or regulated in terms of their health impact by any government agency and can be quite misleading to the consumer. Health-halo items may be loaded with sugar, highly processed oils, or other additives and chemicals. Health-halo foods include:

Flavored waters or sport drinks. These products do contain beneficial electrolytes and vitamins, but they may also include plenty of sugar—as much or more sugar than a sugar-sweetened soda.

Fat-free or reduced-fat products. When the fat is removed, so is the flavor. Texture can suffer, too. Food companies compensate with added sugar, other thickeners, and flavorings. This added sugar or other carbohydrate can be quite substantial. In one instance, a type of low-fat salad dressing contained ten times the amount of sugar compared to the same brand of regular-fat dressing. Low-fat peanut butter may contain a substantial increase in sugar (up to three times as much sugar versus regular-fat products) to compensate for flavor and texture issues related to removing the fat. Just look at the sugar content of low-fat chocolate milk. It may contain up to an additional 14 grams (around 4 tsp) of added sugar in just 1 cup of milk. Enough said. Products may prominently display "fat-free" on the label even if they are naturally low fat or fat free, like fruit, because this has become such a powerful "health" message. Milk, salad dressings, and yogurts commonly display a low-fat or fat-free status as a selling point, but this is not a balanced approach to nutrition. Remember, natural fats are not the enemy; they are part of a healthy diet.

Fruit juice. Orange juice is NOT a health food, nor is any other fruit juice. Once the juice is extracted from the fruit, it is a sugar shot to the bloodstream and acts very much like a soda or other sugary beverage. Cooked (pasteurized) or raw, fruit juice is a dangerous pretender in the health category.

Fruit snacks and roll ups. These little gems are actually candy in disguise. They are made from 100% fruit juice and actually have "bits" of fruit, but this is NOT REAL FRUIT. It is the sugar portion of the fruit without any of the beneficial fiber or other nutrients contained in the whole fruit. This can lead to rapid rises in blood sugar and energy "crashes."

Granola bars or cereals. Some brands are loaded with sugar in addition to the excessive amount of dried fruits. Some contain refined cereal grains like rice puffs. Others add sweetened chocolate, claiming antioxidant benefits. And the ingredient list just keeps getting longer with emulsifiers and processed oils.

Gluten-free. The only people who need to worry about gluten are those with celiac disease or those who have been identified as gluten sensitive. Otherwise, it is not a specific concern. Gluten content has nothing to do with vitamin, mineral or other nutrient content. Gluten is simply a type of protein contained in grains, and different grains contain different types of gluten. There are actually many types of gluten found in all types of grains, but celiac is specific to the alpha-gliaden gluten, and this is the type accounted for on the "gluten-free" label. Most gluten sensitivity is likely to be related to the alpha-gliaden contained in wheat and rye, but sensitivity to the other types of gluten found in other grains can also occur. And yes, individuals who have gluten sensitivity beyond the alpha-gliaden type will have less inflammation and feel better on an entirely grain-free diet, not just the "labeled" gluten-free diet.

Commercial Green Juices or Smoothies do contain green vegetables, but they also contain fruit juices or fruit concentrates in large quantities to sweeten the green juice. Just say no!

Yogurt. Yogurt, especially the prepackaged kid-size yogurt tubes, often contain dyes and sweeteners and may not contain actual live probiotics. Not only are you eating chemical dyes and sugar, but you are NOT getting the health benefits of traditional live yogurt cultures. One popular brand of yogurt contains as much sugar as an 8 oz. bottle of sweetened soda! Also beware of labeling tricks like "Greek-*style* yogurt" vs. "Greek yogurt," known for its higher protein content. The word "style" allows the producer to add other ingredients, and this is not the same as traditional Greek yogurt.

SECTION 4

TOOLS FOR THE JOURNEY TO MAKE CALORIES MATTER

CHAPTER 8

WHAT PROVIDES THE CALORIES IN OUR DIET?

MEET THE MACRONUTRIENTS

MACRONUTRIENTS ARE THE big molecular components of our food. You will recognize them as:

1. Fat
2. Carbohydrate (carbs)
3. Protein

Fiber is also part of the macronutrient family and is considered a carbohydrate.

Macronutrients are consumed in various amounts over the course of a day to give us energy. They provide the calories in our diet. Each of these macronutrients contributes to our well-being. So is there an optimal combination of macronutrients that ensures optimal health? Yes and no. While there is some agreement on optimal macronutrient ranges, there is definitely disagreement as well. It all depends on who makes the recommendations and what health outcome is desired. The most familiar recommendations are those taught to schoolchildren by the United States Department of Agriculture (USDA). The US government has been making dietary recommendations from this department for decades, even though it is not a nutritional science institution. The recommendations are provided by panels of "experts" from various organizations, many who have ties to the food and agricultural industry. It's hardly an unbiased approach for making nutritional recommendations. There are also other research-based recommendations from expert academic nutritional institutions not affiliated with the government or the food and agricultural industries. Recently, more transparency in the form of mandatory disclosure of any corporate affiliations and financial compensation received from these organizations has helped clarify the basis for how some nutritional recommendations may be influenced.

Given the above explanation, it is not surprising that nutritional recommendations from different organizations can be quite different. This is especially true with fat and carbohydrate recommendations. One government recommendation, for example, the USDA's choosemyplate.gov, recommends that protein intake be around 25% of calories, while carbohydrate intake can be anywhere from 45% to 65% of your calories, but fat intake should be held between 20% and 35%. In contrast, compilations of research from respected scientists and universities have found that boosting fat intakes to at least 40% (a common intake prior to 1980) and up to 60%, while lowering carbohydrate intake, can provide optimal health for many individuals and significantly lower diabetes, cardiovascular, and cancer risk.[20] In fact, certain individuals suffering from seizure disorders and diabetics have been shown to benefit from diets that can exceed 70% fat.[21, 22, 23]

Interestingly, the newest US government Dietary Guidelines released in January of 2016 no longer include a dietary limit on cholesterol, although they do still recommend restricting saturated fat.[24] On the other hand, there are credible recommendations from respected academic institutions and researchers that encourage consumption of certain saturated fats (only in the absence of refined carbohydrates) and warn against a fat intake below 30% because it has been associated with compromised nutritional intake of vitamins and minerals in some populations, especially children.[25, 26] A fat intake below 22% of calories in children is associated with less than optimal growth and development.[27, 28]

So how do you know what to eat?

The most important message is this: NEVER completely exclude one of the three macronutrients long term. And recognize that while there are ranges of healthy intakes, there are also limits. Some intake levels simply aren't safe, like excessive carbohydrate intake in a diabetic diet. A lifestyle that completely eliminates or overconsumes one of these macronutrients over a long period of time will cause nutritional problems.

Understanding that different bodies will tolerate different ranges of macronutrients is a good place to begin your health journey. After understanding your current intake, experimentation with different carbohydrate, fat, and protein intakes can help you learn what optimizes your blood chemistry and body function. Refined carbohydrates and processed foods are NEVER the basis of a healthy diet! Some people may need to restrict grains and legumes while others can consume them without problems, but this is not an elimination of carbohydrates, but rather a limitation of one type of carbohydrate. Many people find that when they increase their healthy fat consumption AND reduce their carbohydrate intake (especially refined) while maintaining healthy protein levels, energy increases, weight decreases, and blood test results are optimal. Your body will let you know how a dietary intake is working for you through blood work, waist circumference and fat distribution, energy levels, and feelings of well-being.

CHAPTER 9

FAT IS YOUR FRIEND

WHY FAT?

FAT IS ABSOLUTELY NECESSARY in the diet. It helps us to absorb vitamins A, D, E, and K, and helps make Vitamin D. It also makes hormones, lubricates cells, is part of all cell membranes, and insulates and protects vital organs. Adequate fat in the diet is important for healthy reproduction and brain function, including the prevention and treatment of depression, postpartum depression, and epilepsy. The most obvious benefit we are likely to notice from eating fat is that it contributes to beautiful skin, hair, and nails. It also makes food taste delicious while providing sustained energy so we don't feel weak and hungry. Diets low in fat compromise cell membranes and disrupt cell-to-cell communication. Simply put, low fat consumption compromises brain function, hormone balance, vitamin absorption, and weight management.

There are different types of fats:

1. Saturated (SFA)
2. Monounsaturated (MUFA)
3. Polyunsaturated (PUFA), essential omega-3 and omega-6
4. Trans-fats (TFA), a special type of saturated fat

Here is some basic fat chemistry and physiology (not too much!), and you will be amazed at how quickly you can apply this information. A fat found in food is a collection of triglycerides. Triglycerides are made up of three fatty acids attached to a glycerol molecule "backbone" and can resemble a pitchfork in appearance. Our bodies break down a triglyceride in food into the individual fatty acids (free fatty acids) for use in construction of many different things in the body, including cell membranes and hormones. Fatty acids can also be used when glucose (a type of sugar) is not available from carbohydrates for energy. Our brains can function well using fatty acids as an energy source.

A fatty acid is basically a chain of carbons, hydrogens, and oxygens with an attached weak acid known as a carboxyl group. Fatty-acid chains are identified by the number of carbons (odd or even) and can be short, medium, or long. They can also be identified by whether they possess a single bond between the carbons or double bonds. No double bond means the fatty acid will be saturated. If the chain has only one double bond between any of its carbons, it is monounsaturated. If it has more than one double bond, it is polyunsaturated. This is the basis for how a fat is identified—saturated, monoun-saturated, or polyunsaturated.

The different saturation properties of fatty-acid chains make them "behave" in different ways in our food and ulti-mately in the body. Depending on the amount of saturation, a fat is either solid or liquid at room temperature. Saturated fats are generally solid at room temperature. Unsaturated fats are liquid at room temperature. Fat in food will have both saturated and unsaturated fatty acids, but the fat is identified by the predominant type of fatty acid it contains. This means that most animal fat is likely to be considered a saturated fat even though it also contains some unsaturated fatty-acid mol-ecules. Trans-fats are a special category of saturated fats and will be discussed in a separate section. The level of saturation also affects the stability of a fat. Double bonds (unsaturated) in a fatty acid make it less heat, oxygen, and light stable. The more double bonds a fatty acid has, the more prone it is to oxidation and rancidity. Saturated fats are the most heat-stable fats; polyunsaturated fats are the least heat stable.

Applying heat to a fat can drastically alter its nutritional safety. Heating polyunsaturated fats will produce oxidation and rancidity, even at temperatures at which the oil isn't smoking. Consuming an oxidized or rancid fat will unleash a chain of inflammatory immune reactions in your body that ends with fatty streaks in your arteries, among other problems. It produces toxic products like aldehyde (which interferes with DNA) and formaldehyde, another highly reactive substance. In the typical processed diet, these highly reactive substances are produced at a level likely to have negative effects.[29] This is not a phenomenon reserved for those who consume a large amount of fried foods. It occurs with any ingestion of oxidized oils. The food industry currently uses polyunsaturated vegetable oils to fry food. Think about this the next time you eat a food fried in a polyunsaturated vegetable oil (fries, anyone?).

Ultimately, the type of triglycerides (fat) in the diet will determine the free fatty acids available for the body to use. So our dietary fat will determine the outcome of some important functions and structures in the body. For example, the human brain is made up primarily of fat, around 60%, so having the right types of fats in the diet significantly affects brain structure and function. The myelin sheath surrounding nerve cells is 70% fat and is responsible for cell-to-cell communication, so nerve function depends on the fat in our diet. Our cell membranes also need to move and flex in just the right way in order to assist the proteins within the membranes, and this fluidity depends on the fat in the diet.[30] If we eat a diet high in polyunsaturated oils, our cell membranes may be too floppy; too many trans-fats (saturated fat) will cause rigidity. If a cell membrane is too floppy or fluid, it can be too permeable and allow toxins to enter. If it is too rigid, the membrane prevents access to essential nutrients and prevents signaling between cells. Rigid nerve cells disrupt neurotransmitter binding and signaling, which can ultimately affect the nerve cell's ability to even survive.

We need both saturated and unsaturated fats in our diet, and, fortunately, both saturated and unsaturated fats are found in animal and plant foods. Fat in the diet will provide nine calories/gram in terms of energy, whether saturated or unsaturated. Sources of saturated fats include meats, butter, beef fat, dairy fats, eggs, palm oil, and coconut oil. Plant oils like olive and avocado, and animal fats like lard, chicken, and duck fat also contain some saturated fat, yet they are known as monounsaturated (MUF) because their predominant fatty acid is monounsaturated. Olive oil is probably the most familiar MUF; it is of ancient origin, used for both medicinal and religious purposes and has a long history of safe human consumption. Polyunsaturated oils are found mainly in vegetable oils in the form of seed or nut oils and fish oils. Polyunsaturated oils contain the most double bonds and will oxidize and go rancid much more quickly and at lower temperatures than other fats (not a good thing). Examples of polyunsaturated seed oils are soybean, canola, corn, cottonseed, safflower, and peanut—and constituted up to 8% of all calories consumed in 1999 in America.[31]

A NEW KIND OF FAT [32, 33, 34]
The interesting story behind the polyunsaturated vegetable oils like cottonseed, canola, corn, safflower, and soybean oil is that these oils did not exist as a major consumer food product before the 1900s. Prior to this time, animal fats (saturated) were the predominant fat consumed by humans. However, in the 1860s, enterprising individuals discovered how to reliably extract oil from cottonseeds, a former waste product of the cotton trade, and created a whole new industry. Initially, cottonseed oil was used as lubricant, in fertilizer, and replaced whale oil in lamps, but was NOT considered a food product

since it had a bitter flavor and a cloudy red color. Its low cost was attractive, however, and further processing could remove the objectionable flavor and tamed the red color to light yellow. By the 1880s, unscrupulous food manufacturers would add cottonseed oil to their butter and lard without disclosing the adulteration, fattening their profits. The tame flavor and yellow color also made cottonseed oil perfect for diluting expensive olive oils in an undetectable fashion. Europe (Italy) imported it by the ton. Animal fat still reigned supreme in the American kitchen, yet increasing costs for lard were beginning to influence acceptance of cottonseed oil. Enter an enterprising German chemist, Edwin Kayser, and Procter & Gamble.

THE CREATION OF CRISCO AND THE TYRANNY OF TRANS-FATS

The year was 1907, and Edwin Kayser, a German chemist, had recently patented two hydrogenation processes that made cottonseed oil into a solid fat. Suddenly, a much less expensive ingredient for making soap was available. He contacted Procter & Gamble, a soap manufacturer, and began a partnership that didn't stop with soap. Since this solid cottonseed oil resembled lard in its color and texture, and didn't go rancid, Procter & Gamble quickly realized this could compete with lard in the American kitchen. This new solid fat did not have a specific name to describe its chemical structure or a history of human consumption, but this wasn't felt to be important, since no safety tests were required of a new "food" product. It went straight to market. The product was Crisco.

By 1911, Procter & Gamble would use their marketing prowess, including free cookbooks appealing to the "modern" housewife, to launch Crisco as one of the most profitable food products ever created, changing the dietary-fat staple of America in less than ten years. Eventually, the chemical structure in this new solid fat would be "discovered" and named as trans-fats in 1929, but only after it had already radically changed American fat consumption more than a decade earlier. Natural saturated animal fats had been replaced with a man-made hydrogenated-fat structure identified as trans-fats.

Trans-fats are solid at room temperature and are technically considered saturated since the chemical bonds on the carbon chains are "full" of hydrogens. They are made by adding hydrogens to seed oils in a special chemical process which changes the geometry of the carbon chains to a "trans" configuration and allows the molecules to stack neatly next to each other, turning liquid oil into a solid. Trans-fats look and act very similar to butter, tallow, and lard, and are highly resistant to rancidity. They are also cheap. Cottonseed oil was the first, but soon, other vegetable oils would be hydrogenated—most notably, soybean oil. Soybean oil became the dominant hydrogenated oil after 1960, and Crisco is now mostly hydrogenated soybean oil.

Trans-fats are the darling of the food industry since these fats can extend shelf life, improve texture, and will not negatively impact flavor in foods. These trans-fats are strictly man-made with tightly controlled levels of hydrogenation; food manufacturers can create just the right texture of fat for different applications. Trans-fats are found in margarine, vegetable shortenings (Crisco), some peanut butters and salad dressings, chocolate coatings on candy that won't melt in your hand, and in most commercial baked goods like cookies, cakes, rolls, and snack chips. How much of an impact have these vegetable oils, liquid and hydrogenated, had on our diet since 1911? Americans had consumed more than 18 billion pounds of soybean oil by 2001—greater than 80% of all oils eaten in the United States—and most of it is hydrogenated and, therefore, trans-fats.[35] So does this fat-change matter?

These man-made trans-fats were known to cause metabolic issues as early as 1957, but they are just so handy in the food industry that they continue to dominate as an ingredient in processed food.[36] It is difficult to avoid them if you're buying processed foods. Trans-fats can be recognized by the term "partially hydrogenated vegetable oil" (that is code for this: "I will make you sick with heart disease!"). Read your food labels. It is important to note that there are small amounts of naturally occurring trans-fats in meats such as cattle, sheep, goat, and deer, but these are different from the man-made variety. Naturally occurring trans-fats differ in one double bond that occurs on a different side of the molecule, and this difference is important, since studies have shown that these are largely free of the damaging health effects found in the man-made variety.[37] Man-made trans-fats do raise total cholesterol and triglycerides and are a known cause of heart disease. They should be avoided!

DO ALL SATURATED FATS CAUSE HEART DISEASE?

No! Contrary to popular opinion, naturally occurring saturated fat in the diet is not the cause of heart disease, stroke, or cardiovascular disease. According to an article in the *American Journal of Clinical Nutrition* in 2010:

> *There is insufficient evidence from prospective epidemiologic studies to conclude that dietary saturated fat is associated with an increased risk of CHD, stroke, or CVD.*[38]

So, where did the idea that saturated fats cause heart disease originate? It all began with Ancel Keys, an influential and passionate scientist from the University of Minnesota, who had a strong opinion about saturated fat and heart disease based on a small epidemiological "study" he had conducted on about thirty men on the island of Crete. Using the observation that these men had fewer heart attacks compared to those in six other countries who ate more saturated fat, Keys developed a theory that saturated fat caused heart disease. The interesting thing about this comparison, however, is that there was data available from the World Health Organization for twenty-two countries, not just the six that Keys used; and when all twenty-two countries were included, there was zero correlation between fat in the diet and heart disease. And this lack of correlation in an observational study is powerful—it can prove a lack of causation—which it did in this instance. Yet this did not influence Keys to re-evaluate his theory.

In 1957, Keys began another epidemiological "Seven Countries Study."[39] Again, he carefully selected countries that supported his idea and omitted countries such as France and Switzerland that had high-fat diets and very little heart disease. The careful selection of data also appeared to show that saturated fat (and cholesterol) was strongly associated with and potentially "caused" heart disease. This epidemiological study, in a climate of fear and frustration surrounding the skyrocketing rates of heart disease recorded since the 1940s, became the authority on what caused heart disease and fueled the diet/heart hypothesis. Despite the lack of additional data from clinical trials, an observational study became the basis for the "prudent diet" of the '60s (which maintained fat levels at around 40% but replaced saturated fats and cholesterol with vegetable oils—both liquid and hydrogenated). This eventually led to incriminating almost all fat in the diet and ushered in the 1970s low-fat *Dietary Guidelines* and the low-fat diet craze in the 1980s and '90s.

The *clinical* and epidemiological data since then, collected over decades, now clearly shows that this idea, implicating fat consumption, especially saturated fat, as the cause of heart disease, is not accurate. In fact, dietary saturated fat is actually known to effectively raise *good* HDL cholesterol.[40] Low-fat diets (18–30%) in women and men actually increase the risk for heart disease due to a significant drop in the protective HDL-cholesterol levels, and this drop in HDL is even more pronounced in women and raises the risk even more.[41, 42] Based on this additional data collected with much more robust methodology, there is strong evidence that people who consume lower levels of carbohydrates (especially refined) and higher levels of natural fats (greater than 37% of calories) from nuts, seeds, and plants, and natural saturated fat, especially from pasture-raised (grass-fed) and wild animal sources and their associated products, are most likely to have LDL, HDL, and triglyceride levels at lowest risk for all heart-related ailments versus a low fat diet (18% to 30% of calories).[43]

SATURATED FAT AND CANCER RISK

Even more interesting is the focus of these studies on breast cancer risk in women who participated in these fat-consumption studies. The Nurses Health Study, conducted by Walter Willet at the Harvard School of Public Health, followed 90,000 nurses for five years and found that fat consumption is not positively linked to breast cancer. After fourteen years of continued data collection, the study showed that women who reduced their overall fat consumption had no reduction in risk for breast cancer and that risk actually decreased for those who consumed the highest levels of saturated fat.[44] This lack of association between animal-fat consumption and breast cancer is also supported by a study which looked at nearly 500,000 women in Europe and 40,000 postmeno-pausal women in the US.[45] Beginning in 2010, the USDA and AHA no longer promoted specific targets for fat intakes in their dietary guidelines. Today they acknowledge the ongoing research that is reshaping recommendations about fat, especially saturated-fat, consumption.[46, 47, 48]

Dietary saturated fat alone does not promote heart disease or raise cancer risk. It seems to become problematic only when consumed as part of a diet high in refined carbohydrates. Bring on the butter and eggs, but beware of adding that bagel or donut—a 50/50 mixture of fat and processed carbohydrate!

WHY THE CONFUSION AROUND FAT?

There are many reasons why flawed saturated-fat- and fat-consumption conclusions gained such power in the nutritional recommendations from the 1970s on. The diet/heart hypothesis that high cholesterol and saturated-fat consumption (and eventually all fat) "caused" heart disease was put forward by a handful of influential and charismatic scientists overly eager to explain the rising number of heart attacks in American men in the 1940s. The data was seriously flawed by poor methodology and data corruption, but these scientists secured powerful and interconnected positions on both academic and professional associations and eventually controlled all nutritional research funding and the theories surrounding fat for close to fifty years. Opposing scientific findings by credible colleagues were either ignored or attacked by any means possible. Eventually, obtaining funding for a study that might challenge the original heart/diet hypothesis became impossible. More than one illustrious scientific career was ruined if it was determined by the establishment that an alternative hypothesis was being explored.

The refusal of these nutritional authorities to examine or genuinely discuss all the evidence (clinical and epidemiological) is a tragedy for the health of an entire generation and continues to inflict genuine harm to the health of those who still believe the myth that low-fat/high-carb consumption is heart healthy and that saturated fat is "bad." It is also bad for science. Thankfully the original diet/heart studies are being exposed for the errors or biases they contain. Researchers and industries that controlled the nutritional-information landscape for decades can no longer discredit the clinical data coming forward as a result of a generation living these flawed recommendations. Better methodology, long-term clinical data, and the ability to find the "ignored" and disparaged data that challenged the foregone conclusion about fat being harmful (properly collected by qualified scientists) has finally countered the MYTH that everyone should eat a low-fat diet, eliminate dietary cholesterol, and consume as little saturated fat as possible (replacing saturated fats with man-made poly-unsaturated oils and their associated trans-fats).

WHAT ARE THE OMEGA FATS ALL ABOUT?

There are essential fatty acids, meaning we must consume these for optimal health. Two very important essential fatty acids are:

1. Omega-3
2. Omega-6

If a nutrient is specifically labeled as essential, as in the case of these fatty acids, it means our body cannot make the nutrient, and it MUST be consumed in our diet.

Omega-3 fats are anti-inflammatory. They can help lower risk of coronary artery disease, prevent and treat depression, and improve nerve communication. Omega-3 is good for keeping cell membranes flexible and fluid and has been found to influence brain function. These are found in fish, like salmon, pasture-raised meats, and nuts and seeds.

Omega-6 fats are pro-inflammatory. They are important components in blood clotting and cell membranes. Omega-6 fats are found in abundance in vegetable oils, like corn and soybean oils, butter (except grass-fed), and full-fat dairy, corn-fed meats, nuts, and seeds.

Ideally, a good ratio of omega-3 to omega-6 is around 1:1.[49] However, most Americans are consuming 20 times more omega-6 than omega-3, because we consume a lot of processed foods cooked in corn and soybean oil and corn-fed beef. Omega-3 and omega-6 compete for enzymes in the body to be absorbed. Too much omega-6 pushes out the omega-3s. This is bad news for our heart and brain. It isn't enough to consume the recommended amount of omega-3; you must not overconsume omega-6 from things like chips, fried foods prepared in peanut or corn oil, and large amounts of industrial-farmed cheese and meats.

CHAPTER 10
CARBOHYDRATES COUNT IN DIFFERENT WAYS!

WHY CARBS?

CARBOHYDRATES, OFTEN REFERRED TO as "carbs," are our body's quickest source of energy and will spare proteins and fats as energy sources. Carbs are a source of fuel, in the form of glucose, for the brain. Interestingly, though, carbohydrates are not the only source of glucose in the human diet, since the glycerol from fat and amino acids from protein can both be converted to glucose via the liver and kidneys in a process known as gluconeogenesis. This means that there is **no minimum intake of carbohydrate required for survival.** However, carbohydrate-containing foods are an important source of vitamins, minerals, polyphenols, and fiber that contribute to optimal health and add variety and flexibility to the diet. It would be very difficult (impossible under normal circumstances) to obtain all of the necessary nutrients without foods that contain carbohydrates. So while the actual carbohydrate is not a dietary requirement, other components in carbohydrate-containing foods contribute to optimal health.

Carbohydrates are found in plant foods—fruits, vegetables, grains, nuts, seeds, beans, and legumes. Carbohydrates are described as simple or complex, sugar or starch, or fiber, according to their chemical structure. Understanding the differences in carbohydrates is important to promoting optimal body biochemistry.

SIMPLE AND COMPLEX CARBOHYDRATES

Let's talk sugar. The simplest sugar is a monosaccharide: an individual molecule that requires no further breakdown to be absorbed. There are several monosaccharides. Two familiar monosaccharides are glucose and fructose.

Glucose will raise blood sugar and functions as the primary energy source for cells in both humans and animals. Its potential for a quick uptake into the bloodstream can quickly raise blood sugar. It can also be quickly depleted from the bloodstream and cause a rapid energy crash, leaving you tired and "hangry." Despite being called a "sugar," glucose does not taste extremely sweet on its own.

Fructose, by contrast, is noticeably sweet tasting and is the reason fruit tastes sweet. Fructose will not significantly raise blood-sugar levels but instead goes to the liver to be metabolized. And this can seem like a great advantage if you are worried about blood-sugar levels; however, too much fructose can overwhelm the liver, raise insulin levels indirectly, and promote fatty-liver disease and insulin resistance. Fructose does not contribute to the function of the body since it is not directly utilized as an energy source by the body—it's just sweet.

So how do these simple sugars, known as monosaccharides, appear most often in food? Monosaccharides occur in only small amounts on their own in nature. Instead, they link together and form different chain lengths: disaccharides (2 sugar molecules), oligosaccharides (2–10), and polysaccharides (>10) which may branch out. These chains are known as simple or complex carbohydrates, depending on how many sugars are linked together. A disaccharide is simple, and a polysaccharide is complex.

Table sugar, or sucrose, is an example of a disaccharide. It is considered a simple carbohydrate, since the structure of two sugars can be quickly metabolized. Sucrose is made up of glucose and fructose in equal proportion. Once broken down by the body into its two components, which happens very quickly, it rapidly raises blood sugar and requires immediate attention by the body in the form of an insulin release for the glucose and processing in the liver for the fructose. Other disaccharides are maltose (two glucose units found in corn syrup) and lactose, known as milk sugar (glucose + galactose). These simple carbs are quickly and easily absorbed into the bloodstream. The simple sugars of glucose and fructose, in the form of sucrose, fructose, high-fructose corn syrup, and corn syrup, are of major concern in the American diet since these are the likely sources of added sugar.

When a sugar isn't a simple carbohydrate, it's known as a polysaccharide, or complex carbohydrate. Complex carbohydrates are large linked sugar chains that behave differently in the body due to their structures, even though they are made up of the same monosaccharide building blocks found in simple carbohydrates. Complex carbohydrates are classified as starch or fiber. Both types of complex carbohydrates are found in varying amounts in plant foods like beans, whole grains, potatoes, corn, celery, and apples. Fiber, identified as cellulose and pectin, is tightly-wound chains of glucose linked with other non-digestible sugars, and is a structural part of the rigid plant cells walls. Starch, on the other hand, contains both straight and highly branched chains of pure glucose and is found inside the plant cell.

Once eaten, these starch or fiber chains must be broken down into their individual glucose units before being used by the body. Depending on the branching structures of these chains, breaking them into individual glucose units can be quick, slow, or limited. This determines how quickly the glucose is released into the blood stream and the insulin response. In the case of fiber and straight chain starches, there is little branching and structures are tightly wound or crystallized. Digestion is limited or slow, blood sugar does not spike, insulin levels are moderated, and energy levels are more even over time. The branched starches, however, are more easily accessible to digestive enzymes and can behave more like a simple carbohydrate, especially when heated. These are quickly digested, spiking blood sugar and increasing insulin requirements. For more discussion about how a carbohydrate can effect blood sugar, please refer to the glycemic index and glycemic load explanation in Chapter 5.

HOW CAN A CARBOHYDRATE COUNT?

Energy derived from the digestion of a carbohydrate is 4 calories/gram, so if you eat 10 grams of carbohydrate, it will provide 40 calories. This applies to a simple or a complex carbohydrate; however, there is a special category of carbohydrate that will not contribute calories, despite being a complex carbohydrate, and this is known as fiber.

MEET THE CARBOHYDRATE THAT DOESN'T COUNT: FIBER IS FABULOUS

A non-digestible form of carbohydrate is known as fiber and contributes negligible calories to the diet, since it is not absorbed. The main types of fiber are insoluble, soluble, and resistant starch (RS).

Insoluble:

Insoluble fiber is the bulky cell walls of a plant that can't be digested and won't dissolve in water. Examples are the "strings" in a stalk of celery or the peel of an apple. Insoluble fiber moves mostly intact through the intestines since it can't be broken down by the body and prevents constipation and hemorrhoids. It can act as a barrier, which slows absorption of sugars and fats, reducing risk of type 2 diabetes and cardiovascular disease. It also helps you feel full.

Soluble:

Soluble fiber, on the other hand, dissolves in water and has a more viscous, or thick, gel-like consistency. Examples of food with a significant amount of soluble fiber are oatmeal and beans.

It can soak up sugar and cholesterol in the meal and prevent spikes in blood sugar and reduce LDL cholesterol. It can soak up toxins, ferment and support good bacteria, and lower blood pressure.

Resistant starch:

Resistant starch (RS) is an interesting type of insoluble fiber that has some interesting health benefits for the gut. It occurs naturally in foods but can also be added to foods. Resistant starch is basically an undigested carbohydrate that leaves the small intestine. As a large, undigested molecule, it becomes fermented in the large intestine and acts as a prebiotic by feeding gut bacteria. It is literally food for your gut.

The health benefits of this prebiotic fiber include better bowel function, reduced pH, and the production of short-chain fatty acids, including butyrate, that feed and repair the colon, help with inflammation control, and help prevent colon cancer. Resistant starch reduces the blood-sugar response like the other fibers and does not "count" as a carbohydrate or a calorie in the diet, since it is not digested. It's a really good thing. Resistant starch has been known to help those struggling with irritable bowel syndrome (IBS) and other inflammatory-gut issues.

There are four types of resistant starch. RS1 is found in legumes and beans (cooked and cooled prior to reheating again), nuts, and seeds. RS2 is a type of corn starch known as high amylose. RS3 starch is a retrograded starch that forms when you cook and then chill plain rice, pasta, or potatoes (potato salad). RS4 are man-made chemically modified starches that resist digestion.

HOT POTATO OR COLD POTATO!

When starchy potatoes or rice are hot, the starch is readily broken down and quickly absorbed into the bloodstream, raising blood sugar quickly. But if this same starchy potato or rice is allowed to cool for several hours, the starch undergoes a change and becomes resistant to digestion in the small intestine. It becomes resistant starch, a type of prebiotic fiber. It won't have the same rapid uptake into the bloodstream and will not raise blood sugar the same way. A change in food temperature fundamentally changes how our body responds to the same calorie—welcome to food science!

FINDING FIBER

Raw fruits, raw vegetables, beans and legumes, unprocessed whole grains, and raw nuts and seeds contain fiber, both soluble and insoluble. Meat, dairy, processed-flour products, and fat do not contain fiber, even though meat can be described as fibrous.

Fiber can be altered or destroyed by processing. Processing includes cooking, juicing, grinding, and blending. Grinding or blending affects fiber status by disintegrating the insoluble fiber. Juicing removes insoluble fiber. Cooking will destroy much of food's fiber, so caution must be used in how a food is cooked. Cooling a starchy food for a period of time after cooking can increase resistant-starch content as long as the food is not reheated significantly.

Fiber is an important part of maintaining a healthy gut. Constipation and colitis are common problems when fiber in the diet is inadequate. Most Americans do not have adequate fiber intake, due to a high consumption of processed foods. Adults benefit from a fiber intake of anywhere from 28 to 50 grams/day as a mix of fibers. Fiber contains a negligible amount of calories.

CHAPTER 11

PROTEIN PROVIDES

WHY PROTEIN?

PROTEIN IS IMPORTANT FOR energy, muscle building, wound healing, immune function, cellular repair, skin, hair, and so much more. Unlike carbohydrates, our bodies do have a minimum protein requirement for survival. Actually, our bodies require amino acids, the building blocks of protein. There are twenty different amino acids used in the body, but only nine of these must come from the diet. These are known as essential amino acids and are as follows: histadine, isoleucine, leucine, lysine, methionine, phenylalanine, threonine, tryptophan, and valine. The remaining amino acids can be synthesized in the body.

Protein-containing foods will have the various essential amino acids in various amounts. If a protein contains all nine essential amino acids in adequate amounts, it is described as "complete." If a food is missing or lacking in any of the nine essential amino acids, it is considered an "incomplete protein" or will be identified as "having a limiting amino acid." But this does not mean that an incomplete protein is not a high-quality protein. It simply refers to the absence or less-than-adequate amount of an essential amino acid.

It is not necessary to eat only complete proteins to have adequate amounts of essential amino acids, since a limiting amino acid in one food is easily found in another food. It is also unnecessary to choose or combine foods in the same meal in order to get all nine essential amino acids. The key is making sure to eat from a variety of protein sources, either plant or animal, during the day. Any protein will contain 4 calories per gram of energy.

PROTEIN INTAKE

How much protein is needed? According to the United States DRI (Dietary Reference Intake), the average healthy adult requires a *minimum* of 0.8 grams (g) of protein per kilogram of body weight. This means the average sedentary woman needs *at least* 46 grams per day, while a man needs *at least* 56 grams per day. This intake of 0.8 grams per kilogram of body weight is also an appropriate target for a diabetic. An active non-diabetic individual may require an intake closer to 1.0 g of protein per kilogram of body weight per day. For the athlete, intake between 1.2 g (endurance athletes) or 2.4 g (strength athletes) of protein per kilogram of body weight can be a suitable range. Pregnancy and breastfeeding will increase protein needs to a minimum of 70 grams per day for the average woman. Adequate protein intake can represent anywhere from 10% to 35% of calories, but most individuals should aim to consume, at a minimum, 25% of calories from protein.

Some research suggests that intakes above 1.8 g/kg of body weight be counted as 50% toward carbohydrate intake, because protein intakes beyond this level are prone to induce a process known as gluconeogenesis—the production of glucose from amino acids. This production of glucose from amino acids will raise blood sugar, just like a carbohydrate, so this must be accounted for in the diet. This is also the reason a diabetic must be careful about their protein intake. Protein intake must be "just right" to protect and increase lean body mass (muscle) while not creating fat storage. Muscle wasting may indicate the need for more protein, as will high activity, illness, or injury.

While adequate protein is essential, it is important to appreciate its ability to influence insulin levels. Insulin is required for transporting amino acids into muscle cells, so protein intake will signal an insulin release for this purpose. Although protein does minimally raise glucose levels in the blood, the insulin release in this case is really about amino-acid transport. Insulin will be released according to protein dose and type of protein. For example, whey protein is much more insulinogenic than lean meat. This is important for individuals managing metabolic syndrome or diabetes, since their insulin system is compromised. Protein intake, just like carbohydrate intake, must be accounted for carefully by a diabetic in order to properly metabolize energy.

In addition to raising insulin in healthy individuals, protein also triggers a compensatory release of another hormone, glucagon. Glucagon stimulates the breakdown of glycogen in the liver, releasing the newly freed glucose into the bloodstream to protect against blood sugar dropping too low while insulin transports amino acids and sugars into cells. Additionally, however, glucagon also participates in gluconeogenesis, using amino acids if they are no longer needed for muscle building or repair. Protein, when eaten in excess, will end up being converted to sugar in the bloodstream. Insulin will then transport this sugar into cells, most likely to be stored as fat.[50]

Signs of protein deficiency include edema, poor muscle development, failure-to-thrive in infants, poor immune function and wound healing, and thin and fragile hair. Skin will appear dull. The brain also suffers with insufficient protein and can manifest as nervousness. Exhaustion and dizziness can result from a lack of any of the essential amino acids. Biochemically, a lack of protein will manifest in lab tests on the blood as low serum albumin (protein) and low serum transferrin (iron).

WHOLE FOOD PROTEIN SOURCES
Protein is widely available from both plant and animal sources as both incomplete and complete proteins. Plant foods can be either complete or incomplete proteins. Incomplete plant sources of protein include beans, lentils, legumes, green vegetables, grains, nuts, seeds, and even small amounts in fruit. Plants that are considered complete proteins include edamame (soybean), amaranth, and quinoa. Animal foods are complete proteins. Sources of animal protein include

beef, poultry, seafood, dairy, and eggs. It is important to try to consume wild seafood, pasture- or grass-fed meats, and pasture or free-range eggs, because these types of animal-protein sources will have reduced levels of inflammatory fats and lowered exposure to hormone, antibiotics, and pesticide products.

PROTEIN POWDERS

Protein powders have become a widely available protein option and may be either plant or animal based. Plant powders include soy, pea, rice, and hemp seed. These plant proteins can be mixed to achieve different amino acid blends. Animal sources for protein powders include whey, hydrolyzed beef protein, and casein, and these are considered complete proteins. Protein powders can be used as a convenient option to supplement an otherwise healthy, whole food diet. However, care should be taken due to the density of the protein in these powders; it is easy to overconsume protein in powdered form.

Label reading is important here, as there may be additional additives found in these powders. Another concern is the significant chemical processing that may be used to isolate the proteins from both plant and animal sources. Finally, there are concerns about the presence of heavy metals such as arsenic, lead, cadmium, and mercury found in some whey and casein supplements. There are sources for pure protein powders without additives which are safely processed.

When consuming a protein powder, it is important to account for the mixing liquid or added fruits that may be used to make protein powders palatable. This can significantly raise sugar (carbohydrate) content. In commercial premixed powders, the level of sugars used to sweeten premixed "meal" shakes can be quite high. Read labels on protein drinks to understand what you are consuming in addition to the protein. And remember that adequate protein is readily obtained from whole-food sources.

CHAPTER 12
WHAT DOESN'T PROVIDE CALORIES IN OUR DIET?

MEET THE MICRONUTRIENTS

MICRONUTRIENTS DO NOT PROVIDE any calories in the diet, but their intake is just as important as the intake of calories. Micronutrients include vitamins and minerals that are required by an organism, in very small amounts, to grow and survive. Phytonutrients are also considered micronutrients and include any non-vitamin or mineral substance found in plants. Since micronutrients cannot be produced by the body, they must be consumed in the diet. Fortunately, micronutrients are readily found in whole foods. Sufficient micronutrient intake can be reliably obtained from the diet when a variety of properly prepared foods are regularly consumed.

VITAMINS AND MINERALS

Vitamins are neutral organic compounds, meaning they contain carbon in their chemical structure, while minerals are naturally occurring inorganic elements, meaning they do not contain carbon in their structure and are represented on the periodic table—the same periodic table that is taught in high school chemistry. Their influence on health can be very specific to certain conditions like scurvy, blindness, and pernicious anemia (B12 deficiency that results in lack of red blood cells). One of the biggest roles of vitamins and minerals is the ability to act as a cofactor in hundreds of enzymatic reactions in the body, meaning they help promote healthy chemical reactions in the body. In this process of being a cofactor, vitamins and minerals are transformed and can become more physiologically active or help other nutrients become active and better utilized in the body. Not all vitamins function as cofactors, however. Some function as hormones or antioxidants, or play a role in things like blood coagulation and signaling. Minerals can act as electrolytes when dissolved in water in the body and facilitate muscle and nerve function.

There are many essential vitamins and minerals. Essential vitamins include the range of B vitamins, and vitamins C, D, and K, among many others. Some essential major minerals include calcium, phosphorous, postassium, and sodium, and are needed in large amounts in the body (1000mg/day). Essential trace minerals, of which there are seventy-two, are only needed in small quantities and include iron, zinc, cobalt, copper, and selenium—just to name a few. However, the most crucial micronutrients in public health, according to the World Health Organization, are vitamin A and iron. A lack of vitamin A causes severe visual impairment and blindness, as well as poor immune function with higher risk for contracting and dying from illnesses such as measles and respiratory infections. Iron deficiency, estimated to affect 30% of the world's population, causes anemia, lethargy, impaired physical and cognitive development, increased morbidity (disease) in children, and poor pregnancy outcomes such as higher risk for preterm delivery, low birth weight, and generally compromised health in the baby.

It is interesting to note that the discovery and understanding of the essential role of micronutrients has often come as a result of observing accidental or unintended deficiencies. In early animal studies, rats were being fed a diet that was thought to contain all necessary dietary components that provided calories and hydration: protein, fat, carbohydrates, and inorganic salts and water. But the rats did not thrive, even though they had adequate calories. One researcher learned that if he replaced the water with milk, the rats survived, and that some "unknown substance" contained in the milk was necessary. Other researchers had similar findings with rat studies, but at that time the substances remained unnamed. Eventually, the term "vitamine" was coined in 1911 by biochemist Casmir Funk (1884–1967) to describe these vital "unknown substances" which were originally thought to be amines, molecules that contain an organic functional group.[51] Later, it was discovered that these substances were not exclusively amines, the "e" was dropped, and the term "vitamin" was adopted. Letters were then assigned to identify the various vitamins. Vitamin discovery was not limited to laboratories, however.

British and Japanese sailors were also unwitting participants in vitamin discovery due to deficiency issues known to
develop in the men who took long voyages. Sailors consumed
a more restricted diet and were notoriously plagued with conditions known as beriberi, a vitamin B1 (thiamine) deficiency,
and scurvy, a vitamin C deficiency. When the British navy
discovered that consuming citrus could prevent and cure
scurvy in sailors, lemons became mandatory on naval ships,
and the term "limey" came to mean a British sailor (lemon
and lime were used interchangeably). Beriberi, a thiamine
deficiency causing heart and nervous disorders, was commonly observed in Japanese sailors and was cured by feeding
them increased rations of meat, barley, and fruit. Throughout
history, other "patients" have unwittingly consumed restricted
diets, suffered health problems, and painstakingly helped
"discover" other essential nutrients as doctors recorded these
case histories and shared information with their colleagues.
Today, scientific methods continue to improve our ability to
identify and understand food components, and researchers
continue to compile more specific understanding of nutrients
that the body needs to survive and thrive.

PHYTONUTRIENTS

Phytonutrients, also known as phytochemicals, are non-
vitamin or mineral substances found in plants, and there
are thousands of them. These substances have been found
to protect plants from fungi, insect attack, UV radiation,
and other threats. They also provide an array of colors in
fruits and vegetables and impart smell (garlic). Examples of

phytochemicals are carotenoids, flavonoids, phytoestrogens, and resveratrol. They are found in fruits, vegetables, whole grains, nuts, seeds, and beans and are affected by processing, similar to vitamins. The beautiful colors from blue to yellow to red found in fruits and vegetables are indicators of the presence of phytochemicals, and shopping for color in your diet will provide a rich variety of these substances.

Phytochemicals are not considered essential nutrients in the human diet like vitamins and minerals, but they can have powerful effects on your health. Research has shown that having consistent intake of phytonutrients in the diet can decrease inflammation, assist in optimal function of the body, prevent DNA damage, and protect against degenerative conditions like Alzheimer's, glaucoma, macular degeneration, and heart disease. They can also help protect against cancer. Phytonutrients do not provide calories. Although often marketed in pill form as a supplement, this has not been found to have the same impact as consuming them from a variety of whole foods. It's best to obtain phytonutrients in your diet of whole foods, both cooked and raw.

CHAPTER 13
FEEDING YOUR HEALTH TRANSFORMATION

CLAIMING TRUE HEALTH

HEALTH IS NOT ABOUT A number on a scale or about counting calories and exercising to compensate for overindulging. Health is not found in a pill that treats symptoms related to a deficient lifestyle. Health is about self-care, activity, and recreation that will re-charge the mind and heart. Health is about having healthy boundaries around sleep and gracefully accepting the inevitable stress in life. Health is about properly nourishing our bodies with wholesome foods prepared in healthy ways.

- Eat REAL, unprocessed food.
- Know what you eat, and love what you eat.
- Learn to cook and prepare whole foods.
- Limit intake of added sugars, and know their different names.

- Feast with all of your senses.
- Take time to eat.
- Produce comes in many colors—enjoy them all!
- Variety = vitamins + minerals + other nutrients.
- Be physically active.
- Calories matter, but they don't count…at least not as much as the TYPE of calorie.

MAKING CALORIES MATTER, NOT "COUNT"

Calories do count for supplying basic function and energy, and we need to get enough, but counting calories in an effort to control weight and/or increasing exercise to compensate for the calories in the extra cookie or treat is not the answer to optimal weight management or health. The science has overwhelmingly spoken that beyond understanding the basic range of calorie intake needed to sustain function and energy, rigidly counting daily calories and continually increasing exercise in an effort to control weight does not reliably work in the long term and is not a recipe for health.

Making calories matter, instead of "count," brings empowerment and enjoyment into eating —this most essential of all human experiences—and frees us from the tyranny of the willpower myth, counting every bite, and "eating less and exercising more" with the accompanying feelings of hunger, craving, and deprivation. The answer to optimal energy, function, and weight management is found in focusing on eating the right type of calories from the right type of fats, carbohydrates, and protein, and understanding the proper proportions of these nutrients that suit our physiology, stage of life, and activity level.

Honoring our body's need for nutrients and energy is done by enjoying variety in our food choices. Knowing that protein, fat, and carbohydrates each contribute to our energy and well-being means we need to include all of these in our diet, but we also need to "listen" to our body's signals about how the ratios and types of protein, fat, and carbohydrates we choose to eat are affecting our body. One person may find that they have difficulty with grains as a source of carbohydrate, while someone else may find that grains work well in their diet. Remember, this is not an elimination of carbohydrates—it is a reduction of one TYPE of carbohydrate.

By eating the right types of calories, we are more likely to create a sense of satisfaction that can naturally balance our caloric intake and support our energy needs—without a constant tally of calories running in the brain. Spend your time counting your blessings, not your calories.

Along with knowing the details of our diet, our blood work will also provide important clues about the direction of our health. Ultimately, the presence or absence of disease symptoms will let us know whether our diet is moving us toward a state of health or a state of disease. Many symptoms will resolve with a change in dietary intake, making further medical intervention unnecessary.

CHAPTER 14
CONCLUSION

EATING WELL AND LIVING JOYFULLY

WHILE FOOD CAN BE REDUCED to a molecule that produces calories and provides nutrients, eating food can elevate the body and mind to a higher state of health. Eating wholesome food can bring together our physical and emotional needs, desires, choices, and creativity to celebrate life and bring joy. Eating can physically and emotionally connect us and nourish us as we engage our senses to see, smell, taste, and, finally, consume the life-giving nutrients. We need to eat frequently and intentionally to sustain life and health. It is up to us to embrace this relationship with food, eat to really live, and make our calories matter.

CHAPTER 15

RECIPES FOR SUCCESS

SALAD DRESSINGS ARE EASY AND ESSENTIAL

IN MY EXPERIENCE, one of the challenges of creating a truly healthy and delicious salad is creating a full-fat dressing that promotes maximum vitamin absorption. Commercial dressings often use highly processed vegetable oils and can have large amounts of added sugar, other preservatives, and sodium that make the dressing rather "useless" as a health tool. It's important to know the ingredients in your dressing and make an informed choice.

Here are three types of healthy, full-fat salad dressings that can be made at home in just a few minutes. These can also be taken on the go to use on salads that might otherwise be "ruined" by commercially prepared dressings that contain unhealthy oils and excess sugars.

RANCH-STYLE SALAD DRESSING

This dressing is gluten-, egg-, and dairy-free

Makes 10 servings

Amount: approx. 2½ C dressing

Prep time: 10 minutes Refrigerate: 1 hour

> 1¼ C Raw cashews* or 1 C cashews and ¼ C
> raw sunflower seeds
>
> ¾ C Water (can add more if needed)
>
> ⅓ C Extra virgin olive oil
>
> ¼ C Raw apple cider vinegar with the "mother"
>
> 3 T Fresh lemon juice
>
> 2–3 Garlic cloves
>
> 1 tsp Sea salt
>
> 1 T Onion powder or dried onion (you could
> use fresh onions)
>
> 1 tsp Dried (or fresh) dill weed
>
> *Optional:* other herbs can be added by personal
> preference

*Cashews have the ability to "replace" milk or cream in recipes. Cashews have a natural sweetness than can be tempered by using sunflower seeds to replace some of the cashews. Macadamia nuts can be substituted for the cashews for similar creaminess. Almonds may also be substituted for *some* of the cashews. It's best to "play" with the ratios of nuts and seeds to determine what you like.

Put all ingredients in a high-speed blender, and blend thoroughly (1 minute). Pour into a glass container with a lid and refrigerate for at least an hour to let the flavors blend together. The dressing will be pourable initially but after refrigeration will be thicker, more like a dip, and can be used as a dip. For a pourable salad dressing, simply add more water after refrigeration, and stir to achieve desired consistency. This can be stored in the refrigerator for a week but does not have the same requirement for refrigeration that a dairy-based dressing will.

MUSTARD VINAIGRETTE

Makes 4–5 servings
Prep time: 5 minutes

> ¾ C Extra-virgin olive oil
> ¼ C Red wine vinegar, preferably raw
> 2 tsp Dijon mustard
> ½ tsp Sea salt
> Pepper to taste
> *Optional:* add herbs like rosemary or garlic

Whisk ingredients together in a bowl or place in a glass jar with a lid, and shake vigorously. This is an excellent dressing for a cobb salad, potato salad, or other mixed-green salad. This dressing does not require refrigeration and stores for a week.

ASIAN DRESSING

Makes approximately 1¼ cups
Prep time: 10 minutes

> ¼ C Rice vinegar, unseasoned
> 2 T Soy sauce or shoyu sauce (or use gluten-free tamari)
> 2–3 tsp Toasted sesame oil

Optional: ½ tsp raw honey

1 Garlic clove, minced or chopped

1 T Fresh ginger root, peeled and chopped

1 green onion, sliced (optional)

⅔ C Extra-virgin olive oil

Place ingredients in a pint glass jar with a lid, and shake vigorously. This can be used on a variety of cruciferous Asian-style salads like those sold in convenience packs, but I especially enjoy this on a grated celery root and carrot salad with cilantro and peppers. This can be refrigerated but will need time to "warm up" and liquefy the olive oil before use.

ENDNOTES

1. United Nations General Assembly, GA 11138, Department of Public Information, News and Media Division, New York, Sept 19, 2011.

2. S. Jay Olshansky, Ph.D., Douglas J. Passaro, M.D., Ronald C. Hershow, et al., *Special Report: A potential decline in the life expectancy in the United States in the 21st Century. N Eng J Med*, 2005. 352:1138–1145

3. USDA, Economic Research Service, Food Expenditure Series. Last Updated April 12, 2016. *http://www.ers.usda.gov/data-products/chart-gallery/detail.aspx?chartId=40094&ref=collection&embed=True*

4. Ludwig, DS, Majzoub, JA, Al-Zahrani A, Dallal GE, Blanco I, Roberts, SB. "High glycemic index foods, overeating, and obesity." *Pediatrics* 1999;103(3):E26.

5. *https://www.ams.usda.gov/grades-standards/organic-labeling-standards*

6. Altman, Lawrence K. "Health: In Philadelphia 30 Years Ago, an Eruption of Illness and Fear." *New York Times*. Aug. 1, 2006.

7. "The Scientist and the Stairmaster": *http://nymag.com/ news/sports/38001/*

8. Volk BM, Kunces LJ, Freidenreich DJ, et al., "Effects of step-wise increases in dietary carbohydrate on circulating saturated fatty acids and palmitoleic acid in adults with metabolic syndrome," *PLoS One*. 2014 Nov21; 9(11): e113605.

9. Ameer F, Scanduizzi L, Hasnain S, Kalbacher H, Zaidi N. "De novo lipogenesis in health and disease." *Metabolism.* 2014 Jul;63(7):895–902.

10. Miller M, Stone NJ, Ballantyne C, et al., "Triglycerides and Cardiovascular Disease: a scientific statement from the American Heart Association." *Circulation.* 2011;123:2292–2333.

11. Ostman, E, et al., "Inconsistency between glycemic and insulinemic responses to regular and fermented milk products." *Am J of Clin Nutr* 74, no.1, (2001):96–100.

12. Blood Sugar Test—blood *https://www.nlm.nih.gov/medline plus/ency/article/003482.htm*

13. Holick, Michael F, "Vitamin D status: measurement, interpretation and clinical application." *Annals of epidemiology* 19.2 (2009): 73–78. PMC. Web. 23 Nov. 2016.

14. Linus Pauling Institute: Micronutrient Information Center, Oregon State University. Vitamin D. *http://lpi.oregonstate .edu/mic/vitamins/vitamin-D*

15. Knoblauch, Jessica A, "Some Food Additives Mimic Hormones." Environmental Health News. *Scientific American* March 27, 2009. *http://www.scientificamerican .com/article/food-additives-mimic-hormones/*

16. "Fruit Fiction: Is it blueberry or blue dye?" *Consumer Reports* December 2012. *http://www.consumerreports.org/cro/magazine/2012/12/fruit-fiction-is-it-blueberry-or-blue-dye/index.htm*

17. Bolbotz, Sara, "Sorry, But It Turns Out Your Favorite Blueberries May Be Entirely Fake." *Huffington Post*, Oct 30, 2014. *http://www.huffingtonpost.com/2014/10/29/fake-blueberry-breakfast-foods_n_6016288.html*

18. Jacobsen, Michael F, The Blog: "Trashables: Oscar Meyer's Lunchables are nasty—but the message to kids is worse." *Huffington Po*st, February 20, 2012. *http://www.huffingtonpost.com/michael-f-jacobson/children-nutrition_b_1163253.html*

19. *http://www.lunchablesparents.com/en*

20. Wood RJ, Volek JS, Davis SR, Dell'Ova C, Fernandez ML, "Effects of a carbohydrate-restricted diet on emerging plasma markers for cardiovascular disease." *Nutr Metab* (Lond). 2006 May 4:3:19

21. Carl E Strafstrom, "Dietary Approaches to Epilepsy Treatment: Old and New Options on the Menu," *Epilepsy Currents*, 4, no. 6 (2004): 215–222

22. Sarah A. Kelly and Adam L. Hartman, "Metabolic treatments for intractable epilepsy," *Seminars in Pediatric Neurology*, 18, no. 3 (2011): 179–185.

23. Accurso A, Bernstein RD, Dahlqvist A, et al., "Dietary carbohydrate restriction in type 2 diabetes mellitus and metabolic syndrome: time for a critical appraisal." *Nutr Metab* (Lond). 2008 Apr 8;5:9.

24. *http://health.gov/dietaryguidelines/2015/guidelines/*

25. Eva Obarzanek, et al., "Safety of a fat-reduced diet," *Pediatrics*, 100, no. 1, (1997): 51–59.

26. Theresa A. Nicklas, et al., "Nutrient adequacy of low fat intakes for children: the Bogalusa Heart Study," *Pediatrics* 89, no. 2 (1992): 221–228.

27. Dennis M. Bier, et al., "Summary 1,2,3," *Am J of Clin Nutr* 72, no.5, (2000): 1410s–1413s.

28. Teicholz, Nina, *The Big Fat Surprise*, 2014, Simon and Schuster. New York, NY. p. 158.

29. Teicholz, Nina, *The Big Fat Surprise*, 2014, Simon and Schuster. New York, NY. p. 86.

30. Membrane Structure and Function. *http://www.mhhe.com/biosci/genbio/maderinquiry9/etext/chapt04.pdf*

31. Teicholz, Nina, *The Big Fat Surprise*, 2014, Simon and Schuster. New York, NY. p. 82.

32. *http://www.cottonseedoiltour.com/history/*

33. Jennings, Barbara, "Dr. Otto's Amazing Oil." Fall 2010. Penn State Online Library *http://pubook2.libraries.psu.edu/palitmap/Cottonseed.html*

34. Ramsey, Drew and Graham, Tyler, "How Vegetable Oils Replaced Animal Fats in the American Diet." *The Atlantic.* April 26. 2012. *http://www.theatlantic.com/health/archive/2012/04/how-vegetable-oils-replaced-animal-fats-in-the-american-diet/256155/*

35. Teicholz, Nina, *The Big Fat Surprise*, 2014, Simon and Schuster. New York, NY. p. 238.

36. Teicholz, Nina, *The Big Fat Surprise*, 2014, Simon and Schuster. New York, NY. p. 240.

37. Teicholz, Nina, *The Big Fat Surprise*, 2014, Simon and Schuster. New York, NY. p. 240–241.

38. Siri-Tarino, P.W., et al., "Meta-analysis of prospective cohort studies evaluating the association of saturated fat with cardiovascular disease." *Am J Clin Nutr,* 2010. 91(3): p. 535–46.

39. Keys A, Menotti A, Aravania C, et al., "The Seven Countries Study: 2289 deaths in 15 years." *Prev Med.* 1984;13:141–54.

40. Robert H. Knopp and Barbara M. Retzlaff, "Editorial: Saturated fat prevents coronary artery disease? An American paradox," *Am J of Clin Nutr* 80, no. 5 (2004): 1102–1103.

41. Robert H. Knopp, et al., "One-year effects of increasingly fat-restricted carbohydrate-enriched diets on lipoprotein levels in free-living subjects," *Proceedings for the Society of Experimental Biology and Medicine* 225, no.3 (2000): 191–199.

42. Carolyn E. Walden, et al., "Differential effect of national cholesterol education program (ncep) step ii diet on HDL cholesterol, its subfractions, and apoprotein a-1 levels in hypercholesterolemic women and men after 1 year: the BeFIT study," *Arteriosclerosis, Thrombosis, and Vascular Biology* 20, no. 6 (2000): 1580–1587.

43. Wood RJ, Volek JS, Davis SR, Dell'Ova C, Fernandez ML, "Effects of a carbohydrate-restricted diet on emerging plasma markers for cardiovascular disease," *Nutr Metab* (Lond). 2006 May 4:3:19.

44. Walter C. Willett, et al., "Dietary Fat and the Risk of Breast Cancer," *New England Journal of Medicine* 316, no. 1 (1987): 22–28.

45. Sabina Sieri, et al., "Dietary fat and breast cancer risk in the European prospective investigation into cancer and nutrition," *Am J of Clin Nutr* 88, no. 5 (2008): 1304–1312.

46. USDA/USDHHA, *Dietary Guidelines*, 2010, x.

47. Alice H. Lichtenstein, et al., "Diet and lifestyle recommendations revision 2006," *Circulation* 114, no. 1 (2006): 82–96.

48. German, JB and Dillard, CJ, "Saturated fats: what dietary intake?" *Am J of Clin Nutr* 80 (2004): 550–559.

49. Gupta R, et al., "Serum omega-6/omega-3 ratio and risk markers for cardiovascular disease in an industrial population in Dehli," *Food and Nutrition Sciences* 4 (2013): 94–97.

50. *https://optimisingnutrition.com/2015/06/15/the-blood-glucose-glucagon-and-insulin-response-to-protein/*

51. Rosenfeld, Lois, "Vitamine-vitamin. The Early Years of Discovery." *Clinical Chemistry* 43, no. 4 (1997): 680–685.

ADDITIONAL RESOURCES

Bunt JC, et al., "Acute insulin response is an independent predictor of type 2 diabetes mellitus in individuals with both normal fasting and 2-h plasma glucose concentrations." *Diabetes Metab Res Rev.* 2007 May; 23(4): 304–310.

Crescenzo R, Bianco F, et al., "Increased hepatic de novo lipogenesis and mitochondrial efficiency in a model of obesity induced by diets rich in fructose." *Eur J Nutr.* 2013 Mar;52(2):537–45.

Demers LM, Spencer CA, et al., "Laboratory medicine practice guidelines: laboratory support for the diagnosis of thyroid disease." *National Academy of Clinical Biochemistry* 13 (2002): 35. *https://www.aacc.org/~/media/practice-guidelines/thyroid-disease/thyroid archived2010.pdf?la=en*

Epplein M, Wilkens LR, et al., "Urinary Isothiocyanates; Glutathione S-Transferase M1, T1, and P1 Polymorphisms; and Risk of Colorectal Cancer: The Multiethnic Cohort

Study." *Cancer Epidemiol Biomarkers Prev.* 2009 January; 18(1): 314–320.

Frid AH, et al., "Effect of whey on blood glucose and insulin responses to composite breakfast and lunch meals in type 2 diabetic subjects." *Am J Clin Nutr.* 2005;82:69 –75.

Garber JR, Cobin RH, Gharib H, et al., "ATA/AACE Guidelines: Clinical practice guidelines for hypothyroidism in adults," *Endocr Pract.*18, No. 6 (2012); *https:// www.aace.com/files/final-file-hypo-guidelines.pdf*

Giovannucci E, et al., "Risk factors for prostate cancer incidence and progression in the health professionals: follow-up study." *Int J Cancer.* 2007 October 1; 121(7): 1571–1578.

Gyllenhammer LE, et al., "Modifying Influence of Dietary Sugar in the Relationship Between Cortisol and Visceral Adipose Tissue in Minority Youth." *Obesity (Silver Spring).* 2014 February; 22(2): 474–481.

Hemmingsen B, Lund SS, Gluud C, et al., "Targeting intensive glycemic control versus targeting conventional glycemic control for type 2 diabetes mellitus." *Cochrane Database of Systematic Reviews* 2013, Issue 11. Art. No.: CD008143.

Hoffman JR and Falvo MJ, "Protein—which is best?" Review Article. *Journal of Sports Science and Medicine* (2004) 3, 118–130.

Isganaitis E and Lustig RH, "Fast Food, Central Nervous System Insulin Resistance, and Obesity," *Arterioscler Thromb Vasc Biol.* 2005;25:2451–2462.

Jia X, Zhong L, et al., "Consumption of citrus and cruciferous vegetables with incident type 2 diabetes mellitus based on a meta-analysis of prospective study." *Primary Care Diabetes.* Vol 10, no. 4 (2016): 272–280.

Johnson RK, Appel LJ, Brands M, Howard BV, Lefevre M, Lustig RH, et al., "Dietary sugars intake and cardiovascular health: a scientific statement from the American Heart Association." *Circulation.* 120, no. 11 (2009):1011–20.

Keenan MJ, Zhou J, Hegsted M, Pelkman C, Durham HA, Coulon DB, Martin RJ, "Role of resistant starch in improving gut health, adiposity and insulin resistance," *Advances in Nutrition,* 2015 Mar 13;6(2):198–205.

Ku SK, Sung SH, Choung JJ, et al., "Anti-obesity and anti-diabetic effects of a standardized potato extract in ob/ob mice." *Exp Ther Med.* 2016 Jul;12(1):354–364. Epub 2016 Apr 14.

Ludwig, David, *Always Hungry.* Hachette Book Group, NY: Grand Central Publishing; 2016.

Lustig, Robert H, "Fructose: It's alcohol without the buzz," *Adv. Nutr.* 4: 226–235, 2013.

Lustig, Robert H, *Sugar has 56 Names: A Shopper's Guide.* Penguin and Hudson Street Press, NY. Avery, 2013.

Mietus-Snyder ML, and Lustig RH, "Childhood Obesity: Adrift in the "Limbic Triangle." *Annu. Rev. Med.* 2008. 59:147–62.

Miller M, Stone NJ, et al., "AHA Scientific Statement: Triglycerides and Cardiovascular Disease." *Circulation.* 2011;123:2292–2333.

Novella, Steven, "Evidence in Medicine: Correlation and Causation." *ScienceBasedMedicine.org.* Nov 18, 2009. *https://www.sciencebasedmedicine.org/evidence-in-medicine-correlation-and-causation/*

Nutrition Source. *https://www.hsph.harvard.edu/nutritionsource/what-should-you-eat/vegetables-and-fruits/*

Paz-Filho G, et al., "Leptin therapy, insulin sensitivity, and glucose homeostasis." *Indian J Endocrinol Metab.* 2012 Dec; 16(Suppl 3): S549–S555.

Phytonutrients. *http://nutritionfacts.org/topics/phytonutrients/.*

PMEP. Extoxnet. Pesticide Information Project of Cooperative Extension Offices of Cornell University, Michigan State University, Oregon State University, University of California at Davis. "Epidemiology." September (1993); *http://pmep.cce.cornell.edu/profiles/extoxnet/TIB/epidemiology.html*

Resistant Starch. *https://en.wikipedia.org/wiki/ Resistant_starch*

Ronsivalli, LJ; Vieira, ER, *Elementary Food Science*. 3rd ed. Van Nostrand Reinhold, NY: Avi Books; 1992.

Rosedale, Ron, MD. *http://drrosedale.com/rosedale_ writing#axzz4CGRHOdNz*

Rosedale R, Westman EC, Konhilas JP, "Clinical Experience of a Diet Designed to Reduce Aging." *Journal of Applied Research*. 2009 Vol 9; No.4:159–165.

Softic S, Cohen DE, and Kahn CR, "Role of Dietary Fructose and Hepatic De Novo Lipogenesis in Fatty Liver Disease." *Dig Dis Sci*. 2016 May;61(5):1282–93.

Simopoulos AP, De Meester F, et al., "A Balanced Omega–6/ Omega–3 Fatty Acid Ratio, Cholesterol and Coronary Heart Disease." *World Review of Nutrition and Dietetics*. Vol 100; 2009.

Kahlon, TS, Chui MM, Chapman MH, "Steam cooking significantly improves in vitro bile acid binding of collard greens, kale, mustard greens, broccoli, green bell pepper, and cabbage," *Nutrition Research*. June 2008. Vol 28; no 6:351–357.

Tiecholz, Nina, *The Big Fat Surprise: Why Butter, Meat & Cheese Belong in a Healthy Diet*. Simon & Schuster, NY: Simon & Schuster Paperbacks; 2014.

USDA Average Daily Food Intake Data 2007–2010. Added Sugars. *https://www.ers.usda.gov/data-products/food-consumption-and-nutrient-intakes.aspx*

USDA Policy Memorandum. Genetically Modified Organisms Policy Memo 11–13. Agricultural Marketing Service National Organic Program. April 15, 2011.

Vos MB, Jill L. Kaar JL, et al., "AHA Scientific Statement: Added Sugars and Cardiovascular Disease Risk in Children." *Circulation*. 2016;134.

Weiss R, Bremer A, Lustig RH, "What is metabolic syndrome, and why are children getting it?" *Ann. N.Y. Acad. Sci.* 1281 (2013) 123–140.

Yang G, Gao Y, et al., "Isothiocyanate exposure, glutathione S-transferase polymorphisms, and colorectal cancer risk." *Am J Clin Nutr*. 2010;91:704–11.

Yang Q, Zhang Z, et al., "Added Sugar Intake and Cardiovascular Diseases Mortality Among US Adults." *JAMA Intern Med*. 2014;174(4):516–524

www.glycemicindex.com

www.glycemic.com

SUPPLEMENTAL MATERIAL

BOOK DISCUSSION QUESTIONS:

ARE YOU A TEACHER OR BOOK CLUB discussion leader? This book is an excellent resource for those interested in having a fun yet factually based approach to health and nutrition. I invite you to consider these ideas when discussing *Mission Nutrition: Calories Matter but They Don't Count…At Least Not the Way You Think They Do.*

1. What was your initial reaction to the book? Did it grab you immediately? Do you often read non-fiction, or was this a new experience for you?
2. What is the significance of the title? Why do you think the author chose this title?
3. Have you experienced confusion with diet and nutrition information you've encountered in the past, and did this book offer clarity?
4. Were you reminded of a family food tradition after reading the author's introduction? What is your family's food tradition?

5. How has this book impacted your relationship with food? Can you identify and describe your relationship with food?

6. Did the book change your opinion or perspective about anything? How have your views and thoughts about nutrition, health, food, diet, exercise, and weight changed after reading this book?

7. Did the information feel accessible and useful to you? What information impacted you the most?

8. Did you have a favorite part or passage of the book?

9. Did the structure and style of the book help the author deliver her message?

10. Do you feel encouraged and hopeful about your ability to care for and feed your body since reading this book?

11. Did you learn something radically new about health and nutrition, or did this book serve to reinforce previously held beliefs or ideas?

12. What makes the author credible? How do you evaluate sources for your nutritional advice?

Want to share and connect with others who have read the book? Join the conversation at missionnutritionbook.com.

SUSAN SPEAR, BS FOOD SCIENCE, MS NUTRITION, MH-MASTER HERBALIST

H AVING TRAINED AS A RESEARCHER in multiple scientific disciplines, including Food Science, Nutrition, and Herbal Medicine, Susan's professional experience extends over a broad range of work in education, patient care, and wellness. As both an alumnus of Brigham Young University and Arizona State University, her undergraduate and graduate degrees involved animal research in clinical nutrition and food product development. Her work with individual clients and volunteering as a community nutrition instructor has continued to develop her understanding of individual nutrition needs outside of the research lab. Susan completed her Master Herbalist Certificate in 2013 to expand her expertise and better serve the needs of her clients. Prior to relocating with her family to Arizona in 2014, Susan worked as an adjunct professor in both biology and clinical nutrition at Westminster College in Salt Lake City, Utah. Besides teaching the students, Susan helped develop an experiential nutrition curriculum for the Westminster nursing program and has instructed at the Snowbird Continuing Education Conference for physician assistants and nurse practitioners. She continues to conduct corporate seminars and one-on-one consultations. More recently, Susan posts on nutrition topics and tips for eating well at NutritiousInsight.com. Susan's motto: Eating your way to Healthy!

www.ingramcontent.com/pod-product-compliance
Lightning Source LLC
Chambersburg PA
CBHW070727220326
41598CB00024BA/3338